AGING AND THE MACROECONOMY
LONG-TERM IMPLICATIONS OF AN OLDER POPULATION

Committee on the Long-Run Macroeconomic
Effects of the Aging U.S. Population

Board on Mathematical Sciences and Their Applications
Division on Engineering and Physical Sciences

Committee on Population
Division of Behavioral and Social Sciences and Education

NATIONAL RESEARCH COUNCIL
OF THE NATIONAL ACADEMIES

THE NATIONAL ACADEMIES PRESS
Washington, D.C.
www.nap.edu

THE NATIONAL ACADEMIES PRESS   500 Fifth Street, NW   Washington, DC 20001

NOTICE: The project that is the subject of this report was approved by the Governing Board of the National Research Council, whose members are drawn from the councils of the National Academy of Sciences, the National Academy of Engineering, and the Institute of Medicine. The members of the panel responsible for the report were chosen for their special competences and with regard for appropriate balance.

This study was supported by Contract Grant No. TOS10-C-004 between the National Academy of Sciences and the Department of the Treasury. Any opinions, findings, conclusions, or recommendations expressed in this publication are those of the author(s) and do not necessarily reflect the views of the organizations or agencies that provided support for the project.

International Standard Book Number-13: 978-0-309-26196-8
International Standard Book Number-10: 0-309-26196-1
Library of Congress Control Number: 2012953334

Additional copies of this report are available from the National Academies Press, 500 Fifth Street, NW, Keck 360, Washington, DC 20001; (800) 624-6242 or (202) 334-3313; http://www.nap.edu.

Copyright 2012 by the National Academy of Sciences. All rights reserved.

Printed in the United States of America

Suggested citation: National Research Council. (2012). *Aging and the Macroeconomy. Long-Term Implications of an Older Population.* Committee on the Long-Run Macroeconomic Effects of the Aging U.S. Population. Board on Mathematical Sciences and their Applications, Division on Engineering and Physical Sciences, and Committee on Population, Division of Behavioral and Social Sciences and Education. Washington, D.C.: The National Academies Press.

THE NATIONAL ACADEMIES
Advisers to the Nation on Science, Engineering, and Medicine

The **National Academy of Sciences** is a private, nonprofit, self-perpetuating society of distinguished scholars engaged in scientific and engineering research, dedicated to the furtherance of science and technology and to their use for the general welfare. Upon the authority of the charter granted to it by the Congress in 1863, the Academy has a mandate that requires it to advise the federal government on scientific and technical matters. Dr. Ralph J. Cicerone is president of the National Academy of Sciences.

The **National Academy of Engineering** was established in 1964, under the charter of the National Academy of Sciences, as a parallel organization of outstanding engineers. It is autonomous in its administration and in the selection of its members, sharing with the National Academy of Sciences the responsibility for advising the federal government. The National Academy of Engineering also sponsors engineering programs aimed at meeting national needs, encourages education and research, and recognizes the superior achievements of engineers. Dr. Charles M. Vest is president of the National Academy of Engineering.

The **Institute of Medicine** was established in 1970 by the National Academy of Sciences to secure the services of eminent members of appropriate professions in the examination of policy matters pertaining to the health of the public. The Institute acts under the responsibility given to the National Academy of Sciences by its congressional charter to be an adviser to the federal government and, upon its own initiative, to identify issues of medical care, research, and education. Dr. Harvey V. Fineberg is president of the Institute of Medicine.

The **National Research Council** was organized by the National Academy of Sciences in 1916 to associate the broad community of science and technology with the Academy's purposes of furthering knowledge and advising the federal government. Functioning in accordance with general policies determined by the Academy, the Council has become the principal operating agency of both the National Academy of Sciences and the National Academy of Engineering in providing services to the government, the public, and the scientific and engineering communities. The Council is administered jointly by both Academies and the Institute of Medicine. Dr. Ralph J. Cicerone and Dr. Charles M. Vest are chair and vice chair, respectively, of the National Research Council.

www.national-academies.org

COMMITTEE ON THE LONG-RUN MACROECONOMIC EFFECTS OF THE AGING U.S. POPULATION

RONALD LEE (*Co-chair*), Department of Demography, University of California, Berkeley
ROGER W. FERGUSON, Jr. (*Co-chair*), Chief Executive Officer, TIAA-CREF
ALAN J. AUERBACH, Department of Economics, University of California-Berkeley
AXEL BOERSCH-SUPAN, Mannheim Research Institute for the Economics of Aging, Mannheim University, Germany
JOHN BONGAARTS, Policy Research Division, Population Council
SUSAN M. COLLINS, Gerald R. Ford School of Public Policy, University of Michigan
CHARLES M. LUCAS, Osprey Point Consulting
DEBORAH J. LUCAS, Financial Analysis Division, Congressional Budget Office
OLIVIA S. MITCHELL, Wharton School, University of Pennsylvania
WILLIAM D. NORDHAUS, Department of Economics, Yale University
JAMES M. POTERBA, Department of Economics, Massachusetts Institute of Technology
JOHN W. ROWE, Department of Health Policy and Management, Columbia University
LOUISE M. SHEINER, Federal Reserve Board
DAVID A. WISE, JFK School of Government, Harvard University

Staff

KEVIN KINSELLA, Committee on Population, *Study Director*
BARNEY COHEN, Committee on Population, *Director*
SCOTT WEIDMAN, Board on Mathematical Sciences and Their Applications, *Board Director*
DANIELLE JOHNSON, Committee on Population, *Senior Program Assistant*

Consultants

ROBERT POOL, Digital Pens, LLC
DAVID P. RICHARDSON, TIAA-CREF Institute

BOARD ON MATHEMATICAL SCIENCES AND THEIR APPLICATIONS

C. DAVID LEVERMORE (*Chair*), Department of Mathematics, University of Maryland, College Park
TANYA STYBLO BEDER, SBCC Group, Inc.
PATRICIA FLATLEY BRENNAN, School of Nursing and College of Engineering, University of Wisconsin
GERALD G. BROWN, Operations Research, Naval Postgraduate School
L. ANTHONY COX, JR., President, Cox Associates
BRENDA L. DIETRICH, Business Analytics and Mathematical Sciences, T.J. Watson Research Center, IBM
CONSTANTINE GATSONIS, Center for Statistical Science, Brown University
DARYLL HENDRICKS, Quantitative Risk Control, UBS Investment Bank
KENNETH L. JUDD, The Hoover Institution
DAVID MAIER, Maseeh College of Engineering and Computer Science, Portland State University
JUAN MEZA, School of Natural Science, University of California, Merced
JOHN W. MORGAN, Simons Center for Geometry and Physics, Stony Brook University
VIJAYAN N. NAIR, Department of Statistics, University of Michigan
CLAUDIA NEUHAUSER, Vice Chancellor of Academic Affairs, University of Minnesota, Rochester
J. TINSLEY ODEN, Associate Vice President for Research, University of Texas, Austin
DONALD G. SAARI, Department of Mathematics and Economics, University of California, Irvine
J.B. SILVERS, Weatherhead School of Management, Case Western Reserve University
GEORGE SUGIHARA, Scripps Institution of Oceanography, University of California, San Diego
EVA TARDOS, Department of Computer Science, Cornell University
KAREN VOGTMANN, Department of Mathematics, Cornell University
JAMES C. WILLIAMS, Institute of Geophysics and Planetary Physics, University of California, Los Angeles
BIN YU, Department of Statistics, University of California, Berkeley

Staff

SCOTT WEIDMAN, *Director*

COMMITTEE ON POPULATION

LINDA J. WAITE (*Chair*), Department of Sociology, University of Chicago
CHRISTINE BACHRACH, School of Behavioral and Social Sciences, University of Maryland
JERE BEHRMAN, Department of Economics, University of Pennsylvania
PETER J. DONALDSON, Population Council, New York
KATHLEEN HARRIS, Carolina Population Center, University of North Carolina, Chapel Hill
MARK HAYWARD, Population Research Center, University of Texas, Austin
CHARLES HIRSCHMAN, Department of Sociology, University of Washington
WOLFGANG LUTZ, World Population Program, International Institute for Applied Systems Analysis, Laxenburg, Austria
ROBERT MARE, Department of Sociology, University of California, Los Angeles
SARA McLANAHAN, Center for Research on Child Wellbeing, Princeton University
BARBARA B. TORREY, Independent Consultant, Washington, D.C.
MAXINE WEINSTEIN, Center for Population and Health, Georgetown University
DAVID WEIR, Survey Research Center, Institute for Social Research, University of Michigan
JOHN R. WILMOTH, Department of Demography, University of California, Berkeley

Staff

BARNEY COHEN, *Director*

Foreword

The shifting balance between young and old—in particular, between working-age people and retirees—is forcing governments around the world to rethink or revamp policies and programs that affect many aspects of peoples' lives. In the United States and elsewhere, this has given rise to an increasingly contentious debate about how to address current and looming fiscal deficits associated with various age-related entitlement programs.

The fiscal problems facing our society are daunting. At the same time, it is important to recognize that population aging also will have important effects on the broader economy. We need to better understand how macroeconomic factors—such as savings rates, stock market exposure, productivity, consumption patterns, and global capital flows—react to demographic shifts. These factors must be inputs to any analysis of fiscal health and of the solvency of entitlement programs.

At the request of Congress and with support from the Department of the Treasury and the National Institute on Aging, the National Research Council undertook a study of the long-term macroeconomic challenge facing the United States because of these shifts in demographics. The NRC organized an expert committee spanning a diversity of disciplines in order to enhance the basis for policy decisions and to offer its professional judgment about the key issues for our economic future. The committee worked diligently to forge a consensus under the leadership of its co-chairs, Ronald Lee and Roger Ferguson, Jr. We thank the co-chairs for their leadership and the entire committee for its efforts.

We hope the insights in this report will be widely used to support serious discussion of the urgent aging-related issues confronting our society and of appropriate policy options to ensure the adequacy of retirement income.

Peter Blair
Executive Director
NRC Division on Engineering
   and Physical Sciences

Robert Hauser
Executive Director
NRC Division of Behavioral and
   Social Sciences and Education

Preface

In 2010, Congress asked the National Research Council (NRC), the operating arm of the National Academies, to prepare a report on the long-run macroeconomic effects of the aging U.S. population. In response, the NRC appointed an ad hoc committee, the Committee on the Long-Run Macroeconomic Effects of the Aging U.S. Population, under the auspices of its Board on Mathematical Sciences and their Applications and its Committee on Population. The committee was charged with distilling a large body of academic research and providing a factual foundation for the social and political debates about population aging and its macroeconomic impacts and about appropriate policies regarding public entitlements such as Medicare and Social Security. Given the breadth of the report's focus, it was clear from the outset that the committee did not have the full empirical underpinning needed to address this complex topic. Hence we are grateful to the Division of Behavioral and Social Research, National Institute on Aging, for providing additional project funding to identify key research needs and develop research recommendations.

No committee could perform a task such as this without the assistance and close cooperation of a great many people. We would like to thank, first and foremost, our fellow committee members. Despite having many other responsibilities, members of the committee generously donated their time and expertise to the project. The committee met six times over the course of the project. Members contributed to the study by providing background readings, leading discussions, making presentations, drafting and revising chapters, and critically commenting on the various report drafts. The perspectives that members brought to the table were instrumental in synthesizing ideas throughout the committee process.

Drafting the report was a collaborative enterprise. The committee divided itself into five working groups corresponding to the major substantive content areas—demographic and health trends; labor force participation, productivity, and retirement; saving and retirement security; capital markets and rates of return; and fiscal concerns. Each committee member made significant contributions to the report in at least one of these areas, and many people were involved in a crosscutting manner. We are grateful to a number of people who were not on the committee, including David H. Rehkopf (Department of Medicine, Stanford University) and Nancy E. Adler (Department of Psychiatry, University of California, San Francisco), who worked with committee member John W. Rowe to produce the commissioned paper "Socioeconomic, Racial/Ethnic and Functional Status Impacts on the Future U.S. Workforce," which helped to inform the discussions in Chapters 4 and 5. Special thanks go to Robert Pool (Digital Pens, LLC), who drafted initial versions of several report chapters as well as the Summary. We also are grateful to David P. Richardson (senior economist, TIAA-CREF Institute), who shared his extensive knowledge of public and private pension plans, household financial security, and retirement preparedness throughout the committee deliberations. We likewise extend heartfelt thanks to Gretchen S. Donehower and Carl Boe (Center on the Economics and Demography of Aging, University of California, Berkeley), who generated population projections, analyses, and graphs used in this report, facilitated the transfer of data between committee members, and prepared the documentation in the report Appendix.

This report has been reviewed in draft form by individuals chosen for their diverse perspectives and technical expertise, in accordance with procedures approved by the NRC Report Review Committee. The purpose of this independent review is to provide candid and critical comments that will assist the institution in making its published report as sound as possible and to ensure that the report meets institutional standards for objectivity, evidence, and responsiveness to the study charge. The review comments and draft manuscript remain confidential to protect the integrity of the deliberative process. We thank the following individuals for their review of this report: Henry J. Aaron, The Brookings Institution; Peter A. Diamond, Massachusetts Institute of Technology; Arie Kapteyn, RAND Corporation; Jonathan N. Katz, California Institute of Technology; Alicia H. Munnell, Boston College; J.B. Silvers, Case Western Reserve University; Barbara Boyle Torrey, Independent Consultant; and David R. Weir, University of Michigan. We also thank Kirsten Sampson-Snyder of the NRC Division of Behavioral and Social Sciences and Education and Elizabeth Panos of the

NRC Division on Engineering and Physical Sciences for their coordination of the review process.

Although the reviewers listed above have provided many constructive comments and suggestions, they were not asked to endorse the committee's findings or research recommendations nor did they see the final draft of the report before its release. The review of this report was overseen by Charles F. Manski, Northwestern University, and V. Joseph Hotz, Duke University. Appointed by the National Research Council, they were responsible for making certain that an independent examination of this report was carried out in accordance with institutional procedures and that all review comments were carefully considered. Responsibility for the final content rests entirely with the authoring committee and the institution.

Lastly, we must acknowledge the efforts of several individuals as well as staff of the National Research Council. We thank Lisa Calandra and Loretta Sophocleous of TIAA-CREF, who helped with many tasks involving meeting planning, meeting arrangements, and facilitating communication among committee members. Amanda Volbert (Department of Public Administration and Policy, University of Georgia) and Michael Wodka (Department of Economics, Cornell University) assisted with research and writing for several report topics during NRC internships undertaken in conjunction with the National Academy of Social Insurance. Within the NRC, we are indebted to Danielle Johnson for providing the essential infrastructure for this project. Danielle skillfully and cheerfully handled a plethora of matters during the panel's tenure, with assistance from Jacqui Sovde and Barbara Boyd. Elizabeth Fikre edited the volume and made numerous suggestions for its improvement. Kevin Kinsella, the NRC study director, managed the overall work of the committee, along with Scott Weidman, Director of the Board on Mathematical Sciences and their Applications, and Barney Cohen, Director of the Committee on Population.

> Ronald D. Lee, *Co-chair*
> Roger W. Ferguson, Jr., *Co-chair*
> Committee on the Long-Run Macroeconomic
>   Effects of the Aging U.S. Population

Contents

SUMMARY		1
1	INTRODUCTION	5
2	OVERVIEW	12
3	DEMOGRAPHIC TRENDS	32
4	HEALTH AND DISABILITY IN THE WORKING-AGE AND ELDERLY POPULATIONS	62
5	LABOR FORCE PARTICIPATION AND RETIREMENT	75
6	AGING, PRODUCTIVITY, AND INNOVATION	106
7	SAVING AND RETIREMENT SECURITY	122
8	CAPITAL MARKETS AND RATES OF RETURN	153
9	THE OUTLOOK FOR FISCAL POLICY	174
10	RESEARCH RECOMMENDATIONS	194
REFERENCES		201

APPENDIXES

A   Population and Related Projections Made by the Committee   219
B   Biographical Sketches of Committee Members   232

Summary

The United States is at the start of a major demographic shift. In the coming decades, people aged 65 and over will make up an increasingly large percentage of the population, and the ratio of people over 64 to people aged 20 to 64 will rise by 80 percent. This shift will have broad macroeconomic implications as well as important fiscal consequences for government programs that help support older persons, particularly Social Security, Medicare, and Medicaid. Because population aging is a gradual process, the social and economic challenges that it poses rarely attract the immediate and focused attention of the policy process. Recognizing the need for further attention to these issues, in 2010 the Committee on the Long-Run Macroeconomic Effects of the Aging U.S. Population was organized by the National Research Council to examine the likely long-term macroeconomic effects of the aging U.S. population. This report presents the findings of the committee.

The aging of the U.S. population is the result of two long-term trends. The first is that people are living longer. Fifty years ago, average U.S. life expectancy was 67 years for males and 73 years for females; today, those numbers are 76 and 81. Longer life is to be celebrated, and the discussion of the fiscal challenges that result should not distract from this key point. The second trend is that many couples are choosing to have fewer children and to have those children somewhat later in life relative to previous generations, so birth rates are lower. In 1957, at the height of the post-World War II baby boom, the fertility rate was 3.7 births per woman; the average for 2006-2010 was slightly less than 2.1 births per woman. With people living longer and fewer children being born, it is virtually certain that the population will age substantially in the next few decades. Health at older ages has also improved over the last half century as disability rates have fallen, and many of the additional years that people are living are healthy ones. However, the decline in disability appears to have stopped around 2000, and the future trend is uncertain. Nonetheless, the committee finds there is substantial potential for increased labor force participation at older ages if people so choose. While the baby boom generation, whose oldest members are now at retirement age, has made the phenomenon of population aging more noticeable, the coming demographic transition is not just about the baby boom cohort. It is, fundamentally, about longer-run factors. Population aging is a broad, more pervasive trend that is here to stay.

There is already a very broad consensus that population aging will place fiscal pressure on the major government programs that help support older persons in this country. Social Security, Medicare, and Medicaid are on unsustainable paths, and failure to remedy this situation raises a number of economic risks. Health care costs per eligible person have been growing substantially faster than per capita income for decades, and if this pattern continues, it will interact with population aging to drive up public health care expenditures strongly. Recent reforms attempting to address this problem could lead to fundamental change in the delivery, quality, and cost of care, but their impacts are as yet unclear.

Leaving aside the effects of population aging on government transfer programs, there are also important effects of aging on the nation's economy. If people continue to retire as they do now, population aging means that there will be proportionately fewer people working to support more and more people who are not working. This means that a larger fraction of national output will be diverted to expenditures by the nonworking older population. This diversion will be even larger because there has been a large increase in consumption per older person relative to younger adults, owing in part to rapidly rising public and private expenditures on health care for the elderly. Changes in the age of retirement have been mixed. Although people are living longer and are in better health at older ages, the average retirement age declined by many years during the twentieth century. However, this downward trend stopped and reversed around 1995, and since then the average retirement age has risen about a year and a half, an important trend. All else equal, this diversion of output to the elderly will make it more difficult to raise living standards.

There are four basic approaches for adapting to the new economic landscape created by an aging population, and for providing the resources to support the consumption of households in their later years:

- Workers save more (and consume less) in order to prepare better for their retirements.

- Workers pay higher taxes (and thus consume less) in order to finance benefits for older people.
- Benefits (and thus consumption) for older people are reduced so as to bring them in line with current tax and saving rates.
- People work longer and retire later, raising their earnings and national output.

The fundamental issue that society faces is how to adapt in some or all of these ways to absorb the costs of population aging. Each option has different implications for which generation(s) will bear the costs, or receive the benefits, of an aging population.

Whatever the economic consequences of population aging for the United States, it is important to recognize that the U.S. economy is integrated in the global economy and that population aging is a global, not merely a national, phenomenon. The past 30 years have witnessed important changes in the global economy, with implications for workers' job security, wages, and benefits. Trade and financial flows produce ever closer linkages across nations. Population aging is even more pronounced in most other high-income countries than in the United States and is progressing very quickly in some developing countries, notably China. In analyzing the consequences of population aging in the United States, one must consider them in the broader context of a globalized economy whose populations themselves are rapidly aging.

Many aspects of population aging are difficult to evaluate, in part because the history of the United States and of other developed nations does not provide many episodes of substantial shifts toward an older population. For example, some have suggested that a future labor force that is older on average than today's might be less productive and less innovative. The committee examined this issue and concluded that any such effects are likely to be small. Others have suggested that an older population might invest its assets differently than a younger one, leading to a drop in asset prices. Again, the committee concluded that any such effect would be small. An older population, and one in which individuals expect to live longer in retirement, might accumulate more assets. These assets, when invested, could help enhance productivity and generate asset income and thus improve living standards. However, the committee was unsure how such an increase in private assets holdings would be related to a likely increase in public debt as the population ages. There is a great deal of uncertainty about exactly how these and other factors might interact to affect future standards of living. The committee believes that even with a significantly older population, living standards are likely to keep improving albeit more slowly, and that the impact of an aging population on overall living standards is likely to be modest. This is not to minimize the impact on particular government programs, which will be large.

The living standard of older people depends in part on their prior saving and asset accumulation. Research reviewed by the committee suggests that between one-fifth and two-thirds of the older population have undersaved for retirement, and the committee expects that the elderly will face greater economic difficulties in retirement than they have in the past, a prospect worsened by their poor financial literacy.

While population aging is likely to result in a larger fraction of national output being spent on consumption by older persons, this does not pose an insurmountable challenge provided that sensible policies are implemented with enough lead time to allow companies and households to respond. The ultimate national response will likely involve some combination of major structural changes to Social Security, Medicare, and Medicaid, higher savings rates during working years, and longer working lives. The committee called attention to the cost of delaying our response to population aging. The longer our nation delays making changes to the benefit and tax structures associated with entitlement programs for older individuals, the larger will be the "legacy liability" that will be passed to future generations. The larger this liability, the larger the increase in taxes on future generations of workers, or the reduction in benefits for future generations of retirees, that will be required to restore fiscal balance. Decisions must be made now on how to craft a balanced response.

It became clear during the work of this committee that there are many topics for which more knowledge would help inform the decision-making process. This report offers recommendations for further research in four areas: demographic and health measurement and projections; capacity to work and longer working life; changes in consumption and saving; and modeling efforts and data needs.

1

Introduction

The population of the United States will age substantially over the next four decades owing to the drop in fertility following the baby boom and to steadily rising longevity. Population aging will have profound fiscal effects as well as effects on the broader economy. Although longer life is a highly desirable improvement in human well-being, it also stresses our economic system because older people consume a great deal more than they earn through their market labor. To the extent that people have prepared for this stage of life by earlier saving and accumulation of assets, the problem is reduced, but in fact older people are substantially supported by public transfer programs such as Social Security, Medicare, and Medicaid.

The generation that reached retirement age in the 1970s and 1980s benefited from a number of favorable factors that supported their standard of living in retirement. The coverage rate for defined-benefit pensions, which expanded after the Second World War, was higher than for previous, or subsequent, cohorts. The level of benefits provided by Social Security rose substantially in real terms during the early 1970s. The introduction of Medicare in 1965 reduced the costs of health care for retirees relative to what they might have planned for earlier in their working careers. Real house prices rose sharply during the 1970s and the 1980s, offsetting the poor performance of the U.S. stock market until 1982. And for those whose portfolios included corporate stock, the bull market that began in 1982 and lasted for over two decades helped to boost their postretirement wealth.

Those reaching retirement age in the coming decades will not benefit from the same tailwinds that supported their predecessors and instead will face a number of headwinds. The historically large deficits of the last

3 years, in part caused by efforts to help the economy recover from the deep recession that followed the financial crisis in 2008, have unfortunately coincided with the leading edge of the baby boom generation's retirement. More broadly, the rate of defined-benefit pension coverage is declining. Social Security, Medicare, and Medicaid face long-term fiscal challenges. The taxes that finance these programs must rise, or the benefits they deliver must be trimmed, at least for some households, to preserve long-run fiscal balance. Health care costs that are rising faster than other prices are also raising the burden of out-of-pocket medical care costs. Although the run-up of house prices during the first decade of this century generated large capital gains for many households now approaching retirement, the post-2008 decline in house prices has left many households with much less housing equity than they had expected to have. The weak economy that has followed that global financial crisis has ended many working careers prematurely, while also lowering the value of many other components of household net worth, such as corporate equities. Moreover, the prospective returns on assets such as inflation-indexed bonds suggest that capital market returns may be low for a prolonged period, making it difficult for "near-retirees" to accumulate assets for their later years.

Fortunately, as life expectancy has increased, rates of disability at most ages have fallen, so that older people today are healthier and more vigorous than their counterparts a few decades ago. Unfortunately, the improvement in elders' functional status appears to have leveled off in the past decade, and the future outlook is uncertain. Longer and healthier lives are a great benefit, not in themselves a cost. But it does not follow that these added years of healthy life can all be taken as postretirement leisure; some may have to be devoted to working longer, postponing retirement, or working longer hours before retirement. If they are all taken as leisure, then consumption at all ages must be considerably reduced to pay for these new years of leisure: Either savings or taxes will have to rise.

Longer life is only a part of the story. Lower fertility causes slower population growth, and this is also a major contributor to population aging. It makes younger age groups smaller relative to older ones, so there are fewer young people to support old people through taxes or private transfers.

The shifting balance of older and younger population groups has given rise to an increasingly contentious debate within U.S. society about how to address fiscal deficits. Projected costs of public entitlement programs seem daunting, particularly in the context of economic recession. Much of the debate about Social Security solvency, for example, has focused on financing issues—whether the program should continue to be financed solely through the current pay-as-you-go structure or whether personal accounts or other innovations should be introduced. In 2010, the National Research Council and the National Academy of Public Administration convened an expert committee to look specifically at the nation's fiscal issues. The committee's report, *Choosing the Nation's Fiscal Future*, outlined the long-term challenges of achieving a sustainable national budget and discussed a number of options for government spending and revenue policy that could lead to sustainability.

The fiscal problems facing our society are daunting. At the same time, it is imperative to understand how macroeconomic changes brought about by population aging affect fiscal imbalances. It is useful here to distinguish between the fiscal effects of aging—that is, effects involving changes in government revenues and expenditures driven largely by demographic change—and the macroeconomic effects of aging (see Box 1-1). The latter involve consideration of how factors such as savings rates, stock market exposure, productivity, consumption patterns, and global capital flows react to demographic shifts. These factors must be inputs to any analysis of the solvency of entitlement programs.

It also is important to note that the fiscal situation in the United States depends in no small measure on what happens in the rest of the world. The U.S. economy is integrated in the global economy, and population aging is a global, not merely a national, phenomenon. The last 30 years have witnessed important changes in the global economy with implications for workers' job security, wages, and benefits. Globalization, driven by rapid

---

BOX 1-1
A Macroeconomic Perspective

This report takes a macroeconomic perspective on the ramifications of our aging U.S. population. Macroeconomics focuses on broad overall movements and trends in the economy, as opposed to microeconomics, which focuses on factors that influence decisions made by individual people and businesses. Accordingly, this report's emphasis and its conclusions center on average or aggregate phenomena. The reader who is not familiar with this approach might find some assertions to be nonintuitive. For example, from a macroeconomic perspective one expects the postretirement cohorts of the population to have accumulated more assets than younger cohorts. This reflects the tendency of people to pay off their home mortgages as they age and to set aside resources for retirement, both of which increase their assets. It implies a rosy picture for the older population. However, within the overall older population there will be many individuals who have not accumulated assets for later life, as well as many who are spending down their assets in retirement in ways that they would rather not. Furthermore, the relative well-being of today's older population might be quite different from that of previous and future cohorts. In reporting on aggregate behavior, the committee is identifying a variable (amount of assets) that affects the overall economy but not the very real individual stresses often associated with that variable.

technological change, has radically reduced the need for spatial proximity of companies and consumers and has reshaped the organization, management, and production of companies and industries. Trade and financial flows produce ever closer linkages across nations. In analyzing the consequences of population aging in the United States, one must consider this aging phenomenon in the broader context of a globalized economy. There are likely to be substantial spillover effects of international trends on our country, and global conditions will influence macroeconomic variables.

The goal of this study is to provide a factual foundation for the social and political debates that will intensify. These debates, centered on deficit reduction, will focus heavily on policies involving public entitlements such as Medicare and Social Security. This report will not address the details of entitlement programs, as this has been done at great length elsewhere, nor will it offer specific policy recommendations. Rather, the intent here is to understand the broader and more fundamental factors related to population aging, to clarify policy-relevant issues, and to suggest policy levers that could be useful in designing responses to population aging.

This study will also serve as a springboard for a follow-on project that will incorporate modeling and projections to develop new insights on the long-run macroeconomic effects of the aging U.S. population. Owing to funding and time constraints, the present study was unable to undertake all the analyses that the committee thought were important. For example, it would be useful to more fully explore the interplay between demographic and labor force factors when considering whether an increasing share of what workers produce will have to be diverted to people who are economically inactive. The next study will seek to better characterize the sensitivities of projections and the interactions between macroeconomic variables. It will delve more deeply into how the uncertainties associated with existing demographic forecasts—which are addressed in Chapter 3 of this report—complicate predictions of economic behavior and macroeconomic performance. Presenting the complexity of that interplay in the current report would have required a degree of detail that adds little to its main messages and might interfere with their clarity. The next study will focus in part on intergenerational trade-offs and will generate quantitative illustrations of specific policy choices. It will also identify the most important available policy levers to influence the adequacy of retirement income and, where possible, identify interactions and complementarities among these policy levers.

CHARGE TO THE COMMITTEE

In the context of deep uncertainty about societal responses to shifting demographics, the U.S. Congress asked the National Academies to form a committee to enumerate and describe the broad macroeconomic forces that will affect, and in turn be affected by, an aging U.S. population.[1] The mandate of the Committee on the Long-Run Macroeconomic Effects of the Aging U.S. Population was to construct a foundation upon which Congress can base its policy debates and also attract popular interest and support for the debate process. The committee was asked to consider a large body of academic research and distill it for congressional and public consumption. The committee also was asked to write its report for a general audience rather than an academic one, much in the spirit of the United Kingdom's Pension Commission reports published between 2004 and 2006. Those documents, commonly known as the Turner Commission reports, were designed to reach out to nonspecialist readers and to capture the public imagination. Given the asset losses and economic turmoil of recent years, the hope is that many more people in this country will be more receptive to such a discussion now than they were a decade ago and more engaged in it.

In addition to informing the social and political debate, this report also suggests where additional research on the macroeconomics of aging would be useful. The development of recommendations on research was made in response to a request from the Division of Behavioral and Social Research of the National Institute on Aging (NIA), a cofunder of this report. The NIA leads the federal government in conducting and supporting research on aging and the health and well-being of older people, and the results of this report should serve to inform NIA's strategic research plans to improve our understanding of the consequences of an aging society.

This committee was charged with setting out a framework for evaluating the long-run macroeconomic implications of population aging. Specifically, it was asked to carry out the following tasks:

- Examine the main sources of existing long-run U.S. demographic projections, with particular focus on increasing life expectancy, rising numbers of the "oldest old," trends in fertility and net immigration, and changing dependency ratios.
- Identify the degree of uncertainty associated with existing demographic forecasts and how it complicates predictions of economic behavior and macroeconomic performance.
- Quantify in detail the influence of the baby boom generation on the path and likely end point of long-run trends in dependency ratios.
- Investigate trends in retirement ages and the prospects for people working longer.
- Evaluate the implications of projected demographic changes on American living standards, focusing on factors affecting income security in

---

[1] This study was mandated as part of P.L. 111-117, The Consolidated Appropriations Act for FY2010.

old age such as aggregate demand savings, and investment, how they interact, and the aggregate burden on society across all public and private channels through which transfers flow.
- Investigate the capabilities for government to maintain current levels of publicly funded support for older people.
- Investigate trends in private pension provisions and how those trends might be related to the transition to an older society.
- Investigate what levels of personal savings would be necessary in order for people to sustain their living standards in retirement for various assumptions about retirement ages, health care cost growth, public support for older persons, and the effects of increased national savings on investment returns. Summarize the evidence regarding savings adequacy for different age cohorts. Investigate the impediments to people saving adequate amounts.
- Develop research recommendations that address knowledge gaps and anticipated data needs identified during Committee deliberations and which reflect an understanding of international differences.

ORGANIZATION OF THE REPORT

The report seeks to consider how well prepared we are as a nation for population aging and to discuss the ramifications of underlying trends in demography and health. Because aging of the U.S. population is still largely in the future, the committee was careful to consider how certain we can be about future developments. The committee also considers some possible policy responses to population aging and trade-offs among them.

Chapter 2 has a dual purpose. Because aging has many effects on both the private and public sectors, it is easy to get lost in a mountain of detail and to lose sight of the big picture. Chapter 2 initially provides a framework for thinking about the broad consequences of population aging and the options we have for dealing with changing demographic realities. The chapter also serves to synthesize the committee's deliberations, weaving the main points from subsequent chapters into a coherent whole that summarizes the committee's primary findings.

The demographic trends that give rise to population aging are explained in Chapter 3. Particular attention is given to the debate about the future trajectory of life expectancy in the United States. The population projections of the committee presented in the chapter incorporate assumptions that are somewhat different from those underlying official U.S. government projections. The chapter also illustrates age patterns of consumption and income as a means of understanding why population aging matters to the nation's fiscal health.

Chapters 4 through 8 examine a range of factors that affect the impact of population aging. Changes in the prevalence and severity of functional impairments will have major implications for health care costs, and Chapter 4 considers recent trends in functional status and their relationship to socioeconomic variables and to disability. Chapter 5 examines patterns of labor force participation and retirement, highlights some of the attitudes and institutional features that influence employment behavior, and assesses the macro-level implications of longer working lives. Chapter 6 explores the intersection of population aging, technological innovation, and productivity; discusses what is known about the impact of a changing population age distribution on overall economic productivity; and suggests several pathways from a shifting age distribution to greater productivity and income. Chapter 7 tackles the complex relationship between aging populations and long-run rates of return on investments. The discussion considers various ways in which population aging affects capital markets, and emphasizes the importance of a global perspective. Chapter 8 looks at patterns of saving and wealth in the United States, considers whether saving is likely to be sufficient for future needs, and discusses several approaches to enhancing retirement security.

Chapter 9 examines the impact of population aging on federal and state budgets, noting that the projected imbalances between revenues and expenditures are only partially explained by demographic change. The discussion outlines a strategy for analyzing the macroeconomic effects of a given policy trajectory. The strategy includes estimation of the inter- and intragenerational distribution of changes in resources and marginal tax rates under the policy, the timing of anticipated policy changes, and the possibility of alternative policy paths and how they could impact economic trajectories.

From the committee's deliberations emerged four clusters of topics on which additional research is recommended. The committee hopes these ideas, which are presented in the final chapter, will foster research that can better inform the relationships among the key variables discussed in this report. It hopes as well that such research will translate into macroeconomic modeling that allows us to identify and quantify the potential impact of policy changes on the well-being of the nation and its people.

2

Overview

INTRODUCTION

The United States is undergoing a profound change as the number and fraction of older persons in the population rise. Similar changes are occurring around the world as an inevitable consequence of longer life and fewer births per woman. At the same time, the meaning of chronological age has changed. In terms of health and vitality, many "old" people today are functionally similar to younger persons living a few decades ago. A rising proportion of those in their seventh or eighth decades of life does not necessarily mean that more people are unable to work or care for themselves. In this important sense, the part of population aging due to longer life is not a problem; rather, it reflects revolutionary changes in health and longevity of the population (the part of population aging due to lower birth rates is a different matter).

Nonetheless, many of our policies, institutions, and behaviors are structured by chronological age, with age 65 having played a particularly important role in the last half century or so. If Americans continue to retire around age 65, then longer life and population aging will indeed be costly. As the share of the population 65 and over grows, there will be fewer workers to support them. Although we expect productivity to continue to grow and living standards to rise, if the population does not work longer and retire later, we will have to set aside a greater share of our earnings to provide for old age. Since changing this demographic trend is not a realistic option, we cannot continue our economic behaviors and policies as in the past. We must adjust to the changing demographic realities, including lower birth rates, a workforce that is growing more slowly, and longer lives.

Our options are few: We must consume less, work more, or both. There are four basic approaches for adapting to the new economic landscape created by an aging population, and for providing the resources to support the consumption of households in their later years:

- Workers save more (and consume less) in order to prepare better for their retirements.
- Workers pay higher taxes (and thus consume less) in order to finance benefits for older people.
- Benefits (and thus consumption) for older people are reduced so as to bring them in line with current tax and saving rates.
- People work longer and retire later, raising their earnings and total output.

Higher saving rates for the working age population would reduce their current consumption but enable them to rely less heavily on public benefits for pensions and health care in the future. Of course, higher saving rates for the young will not help pay for the benefits of the current elderly. (For some basic definitions, see Box 2-1.) Raising payroll taxes would reduce consumption by the working age population, making it possible to pay more benefits to the current and future elderly. Alternatively, costs could be shifted to the elderly by cutting their benefits or raising their taxes as a condition for receiving the benefits. A final option is to increase the size of the

---

BOX 2-1
Basic Definitions

There is increasing recognition that the term "elderly" is an inadequate generalization that obscures the diversity of a population age group that spans more than 40 years. Nevertheless, for purposes of comparison—over time, across countries, and sometimes over different variables—some chronological demarcation of age categories is necessary. This report uses the term "elderly" to refer to people aged 65 and over.

The "developed" and "developing" country categories used in this report correspond directly to the "more developed" and "less developed" classification used by the United Nations. Developed countries comprise all nations in Europe (including some nations that were part of the former Soviet Union) and North America, plus Japan, Australia, and New Zealand. The other nations of the world are classified as developing countries. While these two broad categories commonly are used for comparative purposes, it is increasingly evident that they often do not accurately reflect developmental differences between nations.

labor force, possibly by raising labor supply during the traditional working years but more likely by extending time in the labor force and retiring later.

The fundamental issue that society faces is how to allocate the increased costs of population aging across these four sources. Each of the options has different implications for which age groups and which generations will bear the costs and enjoy the benefits. If benefits of the elderly are cut now, then this group will be permanently worse off because they will not recoup this loss in a later period. If, instead, benefits for the elderly are preserved by raising taxes, then current workers will consume less. They may gain later on from the higher benefits once they themselves are old, but how much depends on economic growth. The same will be true of later generations. If we ask current workers to save more, this would help reduce taxes and benefits in the long run, but it will not help pay the rising costs of benefits for the current elderly.

The longer our nation delays making changes to the benefit and tax structures associated with entitlement programs for older individuals, the larger will be the "legacy liability" that will be passed to future generations. The larger this liability, the larger the increase in taxes on future generations of workers, or the reduction in benefits for future generations of retirees, that will be required to restore fiscal balance. The same is true for raising retirement ages. The remaining chapters in this report discuss these and related issues in more depth. The purpose of this chapter is to present a coherent view of the primary findings discussed in the following chapters, where supporting evidence and references may be found.

Of course, population aging has other consequences that are not explicitly addressed in this report. It has many social effects, from impacts on families and household structure through needs for the redesign of transportation networks and the built environment. But here our focus is more narrowly on the long-term consequences for the macroeconomy.

DEMOGRAPHIC CHANGE

Population Aging Is Global

Populations are aging all over the world, but the pace and timing vary by country and region. In the wealthier nations, the aggregate median age has risen from 29 years in 1950 to 39 in 2010 and is projected to reach 48 by 2050. In the developing countries, the median age now is 27, but they too are aging, and their median age is projected to reach 37 by 2050. This aging of populations will influence the U.S. economy through globalized markets for goods, capital, and labor. U.S. wages, profit rates, and capital per worker depend in part on national factors, but also on these international ones. The old age dependency ratio is the ratio of the population aged 65 and above to the population aged 20 to 64.[1] The global old age dependency ratio is currently much lower than in the United States because of the preponderance of less-developed nations in the world population. For international markets, however, levels of income also matter. And when we take gross domestic product (GDP) into account (Chapter 8), the global old age dependency ratio is very similar to that of the United States. Projections suggest that this will remain true through 2050.

On average, people tend to accumulate assets over their lifetimes, and the elderly hold more assets than the young, particularly if we count pension plan assets. For this reason, population aging tends to boost wealth per capita and per worker, perhaps reducing its rate of return. To capture higher returns, investment may flow from older countries to younger ones. Population aging can be expected to alter international capital flows, and the patterns may be complex.

Birth, Mortality, and Population Growth

As mortality rates have fallen in the United States, the average length of life has risen from 47 years in 1900 to 78 today, and it is expected to continue to rise in coming decades. The committee projects U.S. life expectancy to reach 84.5 years by 2050 (Chapter 3). The average person living now is much more likely to survive until age 65 or 70 and to live more years thereafter. This is aging at the level of the individual.

A second and less obvious cause of population aging is a decline in the birth rate. With lower birth rates, younger generations are smaller relative to older generations, and this raises the average age of the population. There is a bulge in the U.S. population resulting from the baby boom generation, people born after the Second World War between 1945 and 1965, when there were three or four births per family on average. The baby boom generation is now beginning to reach age 65; members of this cohort are leaving the labor force and being replaced by smaller cohorts. This shift will mean that the number of retirements will be increasing sharply in the next two decades, just as the number of workers is leveling off. The number of retired persons per working person is expected to rise continuously in the years ahead. In this context, it is important to stress that while the baby boom generation has made the phenomenon of population aging more noticeable, the coming demographic transition is not just about the baby boom cohort—it is fundamentally about longer-run factors. Population aging is a broad, more pervasive trend that is here to stay.

---

[1]This will be the definition throughout the report, unless otherwise noted. The concept is based on chronological age and is subject to the limitations noted earlier in this chapter and elsewhere.

The United States is not alone in experiencing population aging. The entire world has embarked on this journey. The high-income countries are farthest along in the process, but many middle-income and lower-income countries will have slowing growth and aging populations in the coming decades because of their rapid and deep fertility declines. The United States is among the youngest of the rich nations because others generally have lower birth rates and lower immigration rates (immigrants are younger on average than the native-born population). Population aging through 2050 will be relatively modest in the United States compared to that in Japan and European nations.

While the future is uncertain, everyone who will reach age 65 by 2050 has already been born, as have many of the younger people who will be in the workforce then. As discussed in Chapter 3, the ratio of people aged 65 and over to people aged 20-64 will likely rise by 80 percent between now and 2050, and there is only a 1 in 40 chance that the increase will be less than 60 percent. Accordingly, we can be virtually certain that very substantial population aging is going to occur. Given the current age patterns of work and consumption, the biggest growth will be in age groups in which people currently consume a great deal and work very little. A growing fraction of the population will need to live either on its own savings or on public transfers. This is what makes population aging challenging for individuals and for public policy.

Changing Health

An important feature of rising life expectancy concerns the quality of life of the older years. As more people enter their seventh, eighth, and ninth decades, are these years likely to be healthy or unhealthy? Active or disabled? Engaged with family and society, or isolated and depressed?

If rising life expectancy merely added years of unhealthy, disabled, and isolated lives, the aging trend could be viewed with mixed feelings by older individuals and would probably become costly to society at large. Fortunately, the evidence shows that for most people, added years of life are largely active ones. Until very recently, rates of disability at older ages declined along with mortality rates. However, a number of recent studies have found that these declines ceased during the past decade, clouding the prognosis for future improvements in functional impairments.

Regardless of the time trends in disability rates by age, as the population ages, more people will be disabled and in ill health. The characteristics of the adult population will be changing in other ways as well, with a rising proportion of Hispanics and Asians, an increase in the level of education, and growing obesity. Some of these changes in demographic composition will tend to raise disabilities on average, and others to lower them.

How will all these changes affect the ability of the adult population to work in the coming decades? An analysis commissioned by the committee indicates that, taking into account all these changes in the population, the proportion aged 20 to 74 who will be able to work will decline very slightly between now and 2050, from 91 percent to 89 percent (Chapter 5). Most people will have plenty of healthy years still available at the time they retire. Later retirement is both a realistic policy option and an available individual choice.

An important question for individuals and policy makers is whether those who do not work are out of the labor force owing to health impairments or because of a combination of economic forces and personal choices about work and leisure. At present, 83 percent of the population aged 65 and over is not working. Studies reviewed in Chapters 4 and 5 indicate that, although many older people are out of the labor force, this mainly reflects their work-leisure choice and their economic situation rather than a deterioration in their health status. Of those who are out of the labor force in their 60s, the majority do not report having even a minor impairment, let alone a major disability. Even in their early 70s, a substantial fraction of people not in the labor force have no functional impairment.

One of the important implications of these results is that the nation needs to rethink its outlook and policies about working and retirement. In many countries, including the United States, the age of 65 has conventionally been considered the "normal" retirement age, and this chronological age has been incorporated into many public policies and private attitudes. The committee believes that age 65 is an increasingly obsolete threshold for defining old age and for conditioning benefits for the elderly. Trends in education, health, mobility, and physical and mental disability suggest a need to reconceptualize stages of the life span and reconsider notions about work, saving, leisure, and retirement.

The bottom line is that the nation has many good options for responding to population aging. On the whole, America is strong and healthy enough to pay for increased years of consumption through increased years of work, if we so choose. Alternatively, we will be healthy enough to enjoy additional active years of retirement leisure if that is our decision, individually or collectively.

THE CHANGING ECONOMIC LANDSCAPE

As fertility, mortality, and health status have changed over recent decades, so have patterns of economic activity over the life cycle. At the beginning of the twentieth century, life expectancy among men was 47 years, and two-thirds of those who survived to 65 were still working.[2] The average retirement age of men declined steadily during most of the twentieth century, by 10 years or more, while life expectancy rose dramatically and the health of older people improved. In the early 1990s, the average male retirement age leveled off. More recently, the average retirement age has risen for both men and women, although it remains far lower than a century ago. The pattern for women was dramatically different. Starting after the Second World War, women's labor force participation rates rose, from 33 percent to 60 percent in 2000. The net effect of these changes in mortality and labor supply is that in 1962 the ratio of retired years to working years in the individual life cycle was 0.35; by 2010 it was 0.41, and given the committee's projections, it will rise to 0.52 in 2050.

Age patterns of consumption have also changed strikingly since 1960, particularly if we include health care (Chapter 3). In 1960, consumption after age 60 was lower than at younger adult ages. In that era, although government provided some income support, primarily through Social Security, there was very little public provision of health care. Medicare and Medicaid were introduced in the 1960s, and by 1980, the government provided substantial direct support for public and private consumption of food, health care, and other items. By 2007 the age-consumption profile had been radically transformed: The elderly consumed substantially more than younger people. The combination of declining labor earnings at older ages with sharply increasing consumption means that population aging has become more costly, both for individuals and for society as a whole.

ECONOMIC PROSPECTS IN THE COMING YEARS

The central thread of the committee's charge was to evaluate the long-run impacts of the changing demographic structure on America's living standards, with particular attention to issues such as saving, economic growth and productivity, income security in the older ages, and the ability of government to provide current and prospective levels of support for the elderly.

Our work must acknowledge the substantial impact of the recent financial crisis and the subsequent economic downturn. This report was begun during the middle of the worst U.S. business downturn since the 1930s. While the committee was concerned mainly with the long-run impacts of

---

[2]Much of the increase in life expectancy at birth was due to declining infant and child mortality, the effect of which is much like that of higher fertility. Declining mortality at adult ages has a different effect, raising the ratio of years spent in old ages to years spent in working ages, as is discussed in detail in Chapter 3.

demographic changes, it is aware that the recent economic downturn will leave a lasting imprint on America's economic structure. It is likely to raise the federal debt by at least 35 percent of GDP. It may lead to some deterioration in labor market skills and to an increase in the population reliant on public support programs. Accordingly, even if and when the nation has returned to full employment, the scars left by the recession will likely make the transition to a sustainable fiscal future more difficult.[3]

The Macroeconomics of an Aging Population

Disregarding for now business cycle movements and changes in health status, per capita income depends on two factors: average productivity per person employed and the fraction of the population employed. Productivity, measured as net national product per person employed, grew at 1.56 percent per year over the 1960-2010 period. During the same period, workers as a fraction of the population grew at 0.31 percent per year owing to demographic change, a sharp expansion in the supply of women's labor, and changes in the supply of men's labor. Taken together, these generated growth in output per capita of 1.88 percent per year (Table 2-1).

The committee's projections indicate that the fraction of the population in the workforce will decline by about 0.24 percent per year over the period 2010-2030 as the baby boomers retire, and then decline much more slowly at 0.02 percent per year for the next two decades, 2030-2050. Thus, if productivity continues to grow at its recent rate of 1.56 percent per year, output per capita will grow much more slowly, at only 1.32 percent per year, from 2010 to 2030, followed by growth at 1.54 percent from 2030 to 2050. So population aging will tend to slow the growth in income per capita by about 0.55 percentage points per year over the next two decades relative to past growth since 1960. But this calculation reflects only the changes in the labor force as a share of population and ignores the subtler effects of the aging of the labor force itself and the effect of population aging on the consumption side as the proportion of higher-consuming older persons rises.

The weighted support ratio takes into account these additional effects of future population aging. It is the ratio of the hypothetical labor supplied by the population to consumption by the population, assuming that per capita labor income and consumption at each age remain the same as they

---

[3] It is also important to acknowledge the post-2008 decline in housing prices. While the decline has left many households with much lower housing equity than they expected to have, it is not clear whether this will translate into a major long-term macroeconomic effect. Also unclear is whether housing's contribution to personal assets or consumption is changing because of the aging of the U.S. population. The committee does not believe there is evidence that the value of housing will decline because of demographic-related shifts in household composition.

TABLE 2-1 Average Annual Growth Rate in Output and Workers in Three Time Periods

Period	Output per Worker (% per year)	Workers per Population (% per year)	Output per Population (% per year)
1960-2010	1.56	0.31	1.88
2010-2030		−0.24	
2030-2050		−0.02	

SOURCES: Output is net national product from the Bureau of Economic Analysis (BEA). Workers are persons engaged from the BEA. Hours worked per worker are from the Congressional Budget Office (2012, Table 2.3). Labor force and population from projections made by the committee (see Appendix A).

were in 2007, the last precrisis year, while the population age distribution changes as projected[4] (see Chapter 3 and Appendix A for further details).

The projected weighted support ratio falls by 12 percent from 2010 to 2050. Accordingly, if consumers relied solely on labor income, consumption would be 12 percent lower in 2050 (than if there were no population aging) and would therefore decline by 0.33 percent per year over that 40-year period. It is likely that the economy will experience rising productivity during this period. Suppose that productivity growth continues at its average annual rate over the past half century, 1.56 percent. Even with the declining weighted support ratio, consumption would still be expected to rise at around 1.2 percent per year (i.e., 1.56-0.33 percent per year). In other words, the committee expects that average living standards will continue to rise over the coming decades, but that population aging will make the rise somewhat slower than would otherwise be expected.

Viewed in this way, the impact of population aging on consumption looks modest. Employment has grown faster than population over recent decades, but this trend is likely to reverse, and there will be a slower growth in average incomes due to demographic trends. However, there might be other offsetting factors, either positive or negative, that could change the growth in living standards. This report examines these offsetting factors in detail.

It is important to note that while the macroeconomic effects of aging might be modest for the economy as a whole, particular subgroups of the

---

[4]The methods for constructing the age profiles of labor income and consumption are described in Lee and Mason (2011). Labor income is pretax salary and wages, including fringe benefits, plus two-thirds of self-employment income, averaged across all men and women at each age (including zeros). Consumption includes private household consumption expenditures allocated by age, including education, health care, and imputed services of owner-occupied housing. It also includes in-kind public transfers, most importantly public education, Medicare, and Medicaid.

population could be much more vulnerable. For instance if the burden of adjustment were to be targeted on public programs such as Social Security, Medicare, or Medicaid, or if the costs were born largely by workers or largely by retirees, the overall impact would be quite substantial for the subgroup most affected. Similarly, if the economic cost of population aging were to be expressed in terms of cuts in programs such as Social Security, Medicare, or Medicaid, the impact on the elderly would be substantial.

Potential Changes in Productivity as an Offset to Population Aging

Several factors may offset or amplify the decline in the number of workers per capita and the related changes in consumption that are noted above. Such factors could include changes in underlying productivity growth, in labor force behavior, and in government policies including those influencing the growth in public and private health care costs.

Analyses of productivity growth generally separate the determinants of labor productivity growth into (1) those generated by increases in the quantity and quality of inputs and (2) those generated by technological change and other improvements in efficiency.

Changes in Other Inputs to the Production Process

The first factor—increases in productivity due to higher inputs—involves a wide variety of different forces that could be affected by demographic aging. These might include increases in the quantity and quality of private and public capital, changes in net ownership of foreign assets, and improved education, training, and skill of the labor force. Net income will also be influenced by rates of return and levels of risk for both domestic and foreign assets.

One important topic is how population aging might affect total wealth. This includes most significantly the nation's stock of capital: Its homes, factories, equipment, software, and inventories. Additionally, in an increasingly globalized economy, a substantial amount of the nation's wealth and obligations are international. At the end of 2010, America's total wealth (domestic and foreign) was $46.9 trillion, which was 3.6 times its net national product.[5]

Population aging might affect total holdings of wealth, the composition of assets (e.g., houses, consumer durables, and corporate capital), and society's propensity to hold risky assets. Economic theory suggests that

---

[5] Wealth here refers to current-cost fixed assets from the Bureau of Economic Analysis (BEA) plus net investment position at book value from the BEA. This is a slightly different calculation than found in Chapter 7, which uses flow of funds data.

many households accumulate savings for precautionary reasons and for retirement. If the proportion of the population at older ages increases, then if other things are unchanged, an average household will have higher wealth relative to income. For example, given the actual distribution of wealth by age in 2007, the projected population age distribution in 2050 would suggest a substantial 25 percent increase in national net worth per person aged 20-64 through the mechanical effect of population aging alone.[6] In addition, if a longer life span increases the years spent in retirement, then households will need to accumulate more assets to maintain a given standard of living after retirement (abstracting from Social Security), which could further raise national net worth. These two factors (the need to save more for a longer retirement and changes in the age distribution) tend to lead to higher desired wealth holdings relative to income. This could raise asset income and might also raise the productivity of U.S. workers.

One important additional factor in a nation's total wealth holdings is government debt. Private households that buy government bonds view them as part of their wealth holdings, and these bonds may inhibit or crowd out holdings of capital and other assets in their portfolios. To the extent that households in aggregate do not raise their saving to prepare for the increased taxes that are required to pay the interest, government debt can crowd out national wealth. Over the period 2006-2011, the debt-output ratio in the United States rose by over 30 percentage points.[7] If the rising debt reduced capital and other wealth, then national income would be lower by this amount times the rate of return on wealth. While this would be a worrisome development, most of the recent rise in federal debt has been due to the deep recession and steps to stimulate the economic recovery; to date it has not been caused primarily by population aging or by policies related to the elderly population. Going forward, however, population aging will raise substantially the costs of various public programs, including Social Security, Medicare, and Medicaid, under current benefit structures. Depending on the policy response, aging might increase debt, as discussed in a later section of this chapter.

Although analyses of demographic aging often focus on tangible and financial wealth, the impact on human capital should also be noted. Human capital refers to the useful skills of the population acquired through formal and informal education, training, and on-the-job experience. Economic

---

[6]This calculation is based on the distribution of net worth by age group of household head in 2007 and the committee's population age distributions for 2010 through 2050, taking into account household headship rates by age. See Appendix A for sources and details.

[7]Data on debt refer to debt held by the public and are from the Congressional Budget Office (2012). Government debt would be much larger if it included the implicit net liabilities of Medicare and Social Security (see Chapter 9).

studies indicate that human capital is just as important as tangible capital as a driver of economic growth.[8]

Increased investment in the human capital of our children offers several advantages in the context of population aging. Higher educational attainment is associated with longer life, better health throughout life, and less disability in old age. It also raises labor productivity and helps to augment the relatively smaller number of workers with higher quality workers, which also helps to prevent declining returns to capital as populations age. Education also improves financial literacy.

To date there is little research on the impact of aging on investment in human capital. In the past, most human capital was accumulated in the early stages of the life cycle. Both formal education and on-the-job learning are greatest up to 30 years of age. The other important aspect of human capital is that it can serve as a brake on changes in returns on assets. As will be discussed below, slower population growth may lead to a lower rate of return on assets. To the extent that returns on human capital remain high, this will tend to slow the decline in the returns on tangible capital since increased quality of labor would partially offset decreased quantity.

Improved Efficiency and Technology

The second ingredient in productivity growth comes, over the long run, from the generation and diffusion of new scientific, technological, and engineering knowledge as well as other gains in efficiency. Most of the factors at work here operate independently from our nation's demographic structure. However, one age-related driver for technological change and innovation is the tendency for scientific output of innovators in science, engineering, and many other fields to rise steeply in the 20s and 30s, peak in the late 30s or early 40s, and then trail off at older ages. Yet it is the global trends in basic science and invention that increasingly determine a nation's long-run technological competitiveness. While having a young population can help drive invention and innovation, population aging has very little effect on technological change across societies. Other factors such as income levels, education, institutions, and economic incentives to innovate tend to dominate the actual distribution of scientific and technological output.

As the population ages, so does the labor force. Will the aging of the labor force make it less productive? The committee has investigated this possibility (Chapter 6) and concludes that the impact is likely to be very small. While there may be some adverse productivity impact from a rising

---

[8]For example, Barro, Mankiw, and Sala-i-Martin (1995) conclude that human capital accumulation predicted from their model is roughly comparable in size to physical capital accumulation in the United States.

number of older workers, this is likely to be offset by the favorable impact of the decline in inexperienced workers. Taking earnings as an indicator of productivity by age, population aging in the United States will have a negligible effect on average labor productivity in the coming decades. Nonetheless, there are many other potential impacts of a changing age distribution for which empirical evidence is lacking.

ADAPTING TO THE CHANGING DEMOGRAPHIC AND ECONOMIC ENVIRONMENT

The Need for Action Despite the Uncertainty of Projections

This description of the consequences of population aging is based on forecasts of changes between now and 2050. Yet any forecast is subject to uncertainty, as described in detail in Chapter 3. The fact remains, however, that even after taking account of such uncertainty, the old age dependency ratio is virtually certain (97.5 percent probability) to rise by nearly 60 percent between now and 2050. Moreover, the committee stresses that the mere fact that projections are uncertain does not mean that the government should postpone responding to an anticipated fiscal imbalance.[9] Individual taxpayers and beneficiaries are averse to uncertainty, in the sense that they want to avoid the possibility of a future loss even when balanced by the possibility of an equal future gain. In the same way, they would prefer to avoid the risk of larger future benefit cuts or tax increases even if there is an equal possibility that smaller benefit cuts and tax increases will be needed. For this reason, uncertainty means that action should be accelerated rather than delayed, to lessen the likelihood of very large benefit cuts or tax increases in the future. With uncertainty, it is desirable to have a lower debt-to-GDP ratio than we otherwise would, through additional public saving beyond what would be needed to respond to an expected fiscal imbalance. Of course, the desirability of doing this hinges critically on our ability to resist future political pressures to spend any budget surpluses that might accumulate.

At the beginning of the chapter, the committee discussed the four adaptive mechanisms that America might use to deal with an aging population: We can reduce the relative living standards of the elderly, work longer, increase saving while working, and/or transfer more from working ages to the elderly. Each of these mechanisms is discussed in more detail below.

---

[9]The committee refers here to a "fiscal imbalance," though by law benefits cannot exceed accumulated reserves plus current revenues. When it refers to an "imbalance" it means that, according to current projections, revenues plus reserves will be insufficient to pay the currently scheduled level of benefits.

Reducing Consumption of the Elderly

A first policy option would be to reduce people's consumption when old, relative to their earlier years. If household decisions were well informed and made independently, this might happen naturally as people weigh the relative priority of consumption when young versus old. A reweighting of priorities could lead to a reduction in consumption in older years, or to working longer, or to saving more in younger years (thereby reducing consumption in those years). So households themselves might change their life-cycle consumption patterns if they fully anticipate the need to build a nest egg to sustain them over a longer retirement period. A more complex problem has to do with government transfer programs, where adjustments in taxes and benefits paid must take place via the political process. To date it has proven quite difficult for policy makers to achieve political consensus around the question of how to restore the nation's Social Security and Medicare systems to solvency. Yet doing so is essential if the nation is to provide an institutional context in which households can make retirement plans.

Working Longer

Age at retirement is central to population aging and its economic consequences. Raising retirement ages is one key alternative to reducing the consumption of leisure and enhancing people's ability to stretch their assets over their lifetimes. The average retirement age for men declined substantially in the United States throughout most of the twentieth century. Although this trend stopped in the early 1990s and then reversed, men still retire at a much younger age than in the past, despite their better health and much longer life. Women's average age at retirement has moved parallel to men's over recent decades, but it stabilized and began to rise somewhat later. The committee foresees a continued rise in the labor force participation rate of older Americans. Based on evidence reviewed in Chapter 5, the committee concludes that the potential for work is much greater than is reflected by the proportions of elderly actually working.

Health Status and Retirement

On average, Americans today are retiring in much better health than was true three decades ago (Chapter 5). A substantial proportion of older persons who are not working have no major impairment to their health status. This suggests that, if people choose to work longer for either economic reasons or because of personal preferences, their health status will mostly not be an obstacle. Further, changes in job mix coupled with a general decrease in the physical demands of most jobs bode well for continued labor force participation at older ages.

Will There Be Enough Jobs for the Young If People Work Longer?

Some have expressed concern that if older members of the population work longer, they will take jobs away from the young. Yet this did not happen in the past nor has it occurred in other nations (Chapter 5). The committee thus concludes this is not a substantive concern for the United States in the future. In normal times, except for deep business cycle recessions, the overall number of jobs is determined primarily by the size of the labor force. If anything, an increase in older workers is predicted to slightly increase the wage rates of young workers.

Are Current Workers Saving Adequately for Retirement?

With a larger number of people in retirement and living longer, it would be useful to determine whether they will have adequate living standards during their retirement years. Over the last half-century, much of the worst poverty among the elderly has been reduced, in part owing to government transfer programs. Using updated measures, the poverty rate of the elderly is similar to that of the rest of the population;[10] it is much below that of the nonelderly if in-kind government transfers (such as Medicare) are taken into account.

Looking prospectively, the committee has considered whether saving during the worklife will be sufficient to support an adequate living standard in retirement, taking into account expected future government benefits. This question raises several issues concerning the structure of saving (particularly the changing nature of employer-sponsored pension plans), the rate of return on pension savings, and the prospective impact of demographic aging on rates of return.

Changing Nature of Pension Plans

About half of the U.S. workforce is covered by an employer-sponsored retirement plan, and this has been true for the last half-century. But the structure of pension plans has changed dramatically over this time. In the 1970s, most employer-sponsored pension plans were of the defined benefit (DB) variety, where payouts were based on an employee's earnings history,

---

[10]The standard poverty measure shows lower poverty rates among the elderly, but the new Census Bureau Supplemental measure makes several adjustments that change the picture completely (see Short, 2011).

length of service, and retirement age. Initially, defined benefits were mainly paid in the form of lifetime annuities (though more recently lump sums have in some circumstances been permitted). Capital market risk in DB plans is primarily borne by the plan sponsors, though the participants bear some of that risk if an employer files for bankruptcy and the plan is so underfunded that the reinsurer cannot guarantee full benefits. Today, employer plans in the corporate sector have mostly converted to defined contribution (DC) pensions (e.g., 401(k) or 403(b) plans). Participants must generally decide how much to contribute (sometimes with an employer match) and where to invest the funds, thus bearing capital market risk more directly. At retirement, the benefits are usually paid out as a lump sum rather than as a life-long benefit stream.

The changing nature of pensions has several implications. One is that, in DC plans, individuals may have difficulty determining whether their saving is adequate for their retirement needs. Another is that investment decisions have been shifted to participants who may be unable or unwilling to make informed investment choices. And in DC plans, most individuals are faced with the difficult decision of whether and how to annuitize their assets upon retirement, which traditionally was not the case in DB plans.

In the context of the macroeconomic impacts of aging, a key feature of the movement to DC plans has to do with different incentives to retire. While DB plans traditionally embedded strong incentives for people to retire early, there is no such encouragement in most DC plans. The increased prevalence of DC plans is perhaps the main reason for the increase in the labor force participation rate of older workers since the mid-1990s.

Changing Rates of Return

Some analysts have raised concerns that an aging population will reduce future rates of return or reduce the price of assets, a topic investigated in Chapter 8. The committee concludes that rates of return on investment are likely to have only modest effects on most retirees' financial status because their asset holdings are small, though rates of return will influence savings adequacy for those with greater assets. There are a number of ways that population aging might affect asset returns and prices. Population aging will likely lead to higher U.S. wealth holdings per capita and per worker, which could drive down average returns on capital. Projections of global population aging suggest that these trends will be similar around the world. But population aging could also lead to increased government debt, which would tend to raise returns to capital. Globalization of financial markets implies that broader forces—particularly the overall macroeconomic environment, the business cycle, shifts in global savings and investment patterns, and the rise of high-savings countries such as China—are likely to dominate the pattern of capital market returns in the coming years. Compared to these broader forces, the effects of U.S. population aging on rates of return are likely to be very small. Though major changes in asset prices have occurred and are likely to occur in the future, demographic forces are generally too predictable and move too slowly to cause major financial market dislocations such as those of the 2007-2009 period.

Overall Adequacy of Consumption in Retirement Years

Studies of U.S. retirement saving adequacy produce different answers depending on the methods used, with research suggesting that between one-fifth and two-thirds of the older population have undersaved for retirement (see Chapter 7). Some common themes emerge. First, there is good evidence indicating that low- and lower-middle-income households accumulate few financial and pension assets for retirement. For those households, Social Security, Medicare, and Medicaid are a central part of maintaining retirement living standards. To the extent that benefits paid by these government programs might be reduced in the future, the living standards of the affected retiree households will fall.

Second, the quality of financial decisions, and therefore financial literacy, will play an increasingly important role in how well households fare in their retirement years, particularly in light of the continued trend to DC pensions. Households will need to decide how much more to save and how to structure their portfolios during their working years. They will need to decide when it is economically prudent to retire, taking into account personal, macroeconomic, and political uncertainties. When they do retire, they will need to decide whether to annuitize their accumulations and, if so, how much and with what annuity options. The many households whose wealth rests mainly in their home ownership will need to decide whether and how to use those assets to finance retirement consumption. These are very complicated questions, and financial professionals give varying advice. The committee is concerned that our nation is poorly prepared to move into this changed financial landscape, and it finds substantial value in boosting financial literacy.

The committee concludes that Americans are likely to face greater economic difficulties in retirement than they did in the recent past. Retirement insecurity and saving inadequacy are likely to increase rather than recede, and these will be exacerbated by the need to navigate a more complex financial and macroeconomic structure.[11]

---

[11]It is useful to note that the meaning of retirement has changed over time, and that what might be regarded today as a problem or potential problem (e.g., too extended a retirement, too much retirement consumption, and difficult financial choices in old age) evolved from

While future uncertainties are large, there are many ways to improve Americans' retirement security. These include encouraging people to work longer, raising retirement ages, improving insurance protection and long-term care, and putting Social Security and Medicare on a sound long-term footing. Additionally, while financial innovation has been rapid in some areas, it has been relatively slow to develop products that will help most households manage their savings and transition to retirement. The nation needs to improve private-market solutions such as more saving, better financial literacy, and enhanced financial, long-term care, and annuity products.

Changing Public Policies and Transfer Programs

As noted earlier, the committee concludes that the overall macroeconomic consequences of population aging in the United States are likely to be modest. However, because the government plays a particularly important role in financing consumption and health care for the elderly, many of the consequences of population aging will be focused on specific government programs rather than spread across the economy. For these programs, population aging will have a major effect on costs. Population aging already has led to projected shortfalls in the finances of Social Security, Medicare, and Medicaid and is likely to lead to increasing government budget deficits in the future (Chapter 9). The consequences for Social Security are predictable, and they can be relatively easily addressed by benefit formula changes and increases in contributions. Programs providing health care and long-term care, notably Medicare and Medicaid, are a different matter. Health care costs per eligible person have been growing substantially faster than per capita income for decades, and if this pattern continues, it will interact with population aging to drive up public health care expenditures substantially. Recent reforms have attempted to address this problem and could lead to fundamental change in delivery, quality, and cost of care, but their impacts are as yet unclear.

Government programs are particularly important because it is largely through them that policies could influence retirement ages and perhaps also employers' demand for older workers. Moreover, they could alter changes in consumption for both workers and the elderly. Changes to these programs will also go far in determining how the costs of population aging will be shared across generations and age groups in the future. A critical need in the near future is to put Social Security and government health programs on a secure footing and to reduce uncertainty and mistrust by announcing

---

something radically different. For insightful studies of the history of retirement, see Costa (1998) and Haber and Gratton (1994).

future changes well in advance so that people can structure their plans accordingly. Additionally, policies need to be developed that encourage better adaptive behavior on the part of workers and companies.

Aside from transfer programs, many other public programs could help smooth the transition to an aging society. For instance, programs that make the workplace friendlier for older workers might encourage them to stay at work or to take part-time employment (Chapter 5). Much analysis remains to be done to develop financial instruments such as improved reverse mortgages as well as better long-term care and annuity products. And not least, the nation will need to find ways to improve financial literacy for people who increasingly will manage their own retirement finances from the first days of joining the labor force to the later days of deciding how and when to spend money in retirement.

SUMMARY

The main message of this report is that the committee sees population aging as posing serious but not insurmountable challenges for the United States. From an economic point of view, a larger fraction of national output will need to be spent on consumption by the elderly. Yet an aging population also offers many opportunities, as long as sensible policies can be implemented with some lead time to allow companies and households to respond.

The committee has outlined several ways that the nation could adapt and adjust to the changing demographic structure. Encouraging later retirement is one useful route. It is unlikely to be hindered by poor health or disability. Such a trend could be helped through changes in the structure of pension and health programs and through a continued shift toward DC plans.

Additionally, public policies could facilitate greater saving during the working years as well as provide better financial instruments to turn financial and housing assets into income streams that protect people against the vagaries of longevity. Improving the nation's financial literacy will also be critical in a world where people face a larger number and more complex array of choices about working, saving, and retirement.

Moreover, because of the prospect for a sharply rising federal debt, the nation will need to balance the priorities of different programs as well as provide additional revenue streams devoted to programs for the elderly. There is little doubt that there will need to be major changes in the structure of federal programs, particularly for health.

The committee concludes that our nation must take action soon, rather than simply continuing with the same policies and practices as in the past. Population aging, unlike other aspects of the future, is a certainty, and many adjustments will have to be made. No single feasible policy adjustment is likely to be an acceptable or a sufficient response to the challenge and opportunity of population aging. An aging society need not have lower living standards, slower growth in innovation and productivity, or inefficiently high tax rates. But delaying decisions on how to adapt to our aging demographic structure will make the transition more difficult and costly.

3

Demographic Trends

Around the world populations are aging. This is a relatively new demographic phenomenon because for most of human history populations were young and lives were short. Population aging is largely caused by two demographic trends. Most obviously, people today are living longer than before. A second and less obvious cause of population aging is a decline in the birth rate. With lower birth rates, younger generations are smaller relative to older generations, thus raising the average age of the population. There are other demographic processes that affect aging, including migration, but they generally play a smaller role.

This chapter will examine these trends in the United States, starting with improvements in life expectancy and their implications for the individual life cycle. Later sections of the chapter will discuss population aging and why it matters.

LIFE EXPECTANCY AND THE INDIVIDUAL LIFE CYCLE

Life Expectancy at Birth

U.S. life expectancy at birth started improving in the eighteenth century, reaching 47.3 years in 1900, 68.4 years in 1950, and 78.2 in 2010 (Arias, 2011; Board of Trustees, Federal Old-Age and Survivors Insurance and Federal Disability Insurance Trust Funds, 2011). Increases were most rapid in the first half of the twentieth century, when infectious diseases were brought under control, greatly improving survival of children. In contrast, increases in life expectancy since 1950 have been due mostly to declines in adult mortality as cardiovascular disease became more manageable. The rise of 9.3 years in the United States between 1950 and 2006 was substantial, but most other countries in the world achieved more rapid improvements over the same period. Figure 3-1 compares trends in life expectancy for the United States (black line) and eight other large high-income countries (Australia,

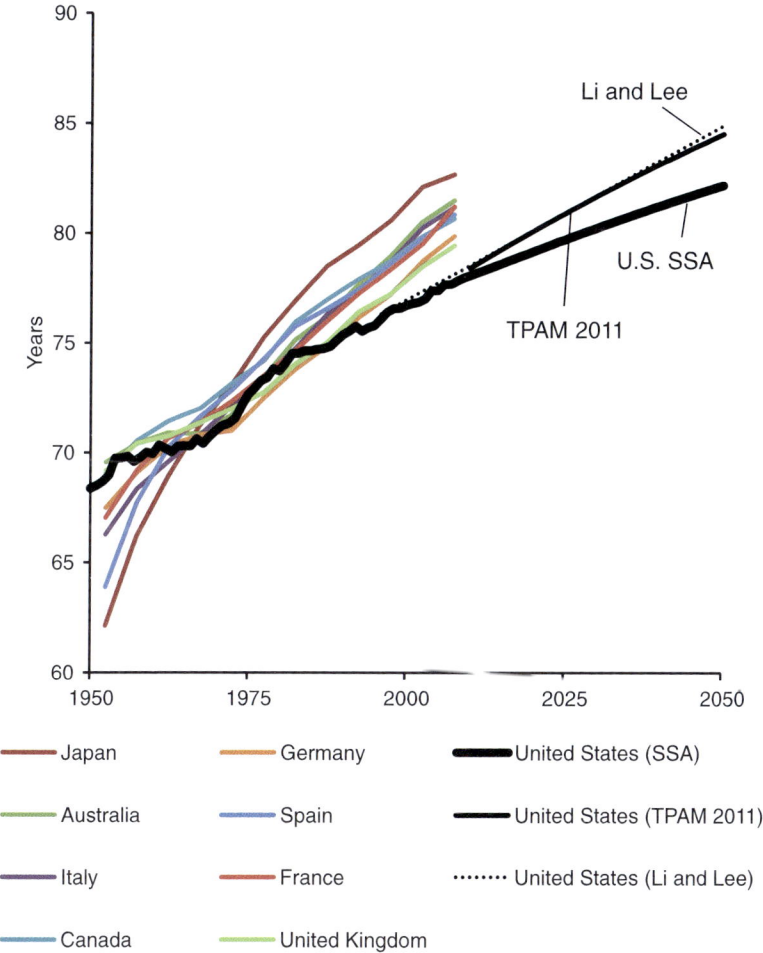

FIGURE 3-1 Life expectancy at birth in selected countries, and alternative projections for the United States to 2050. SOURCES: United Nations (2011); Board of Trustees, Federal Old-Age and Survivors Insurance and Federal Disability Insurance Trust Funds (2011); Li and Lee (2005); and Technical Panel on Assumptions and Methods (2011).

Canada, France, Germany, Italy, Japan, Spain, and the United Kingdom). The United States ranked at the top of this group of countries in 1950 but dropped to last place in 2006 (United Nations, 2011).

Why does the United States now rank so low in international life expectancy comparisons? This question has drawn the attention and concern of researchers and policy makers. The current situation is especially surprising given that the United States spends far more on health care than any other country. In response to these concerns, the National Research Council (NRC) appointed a committee of experts in 2008 to investigate the reasons for this divergence between the United States and other high-income countries. In its final report the committee reached several conclusions (National Research Council, 2011):

> A history of heavy smoking and current levels of obesity are playing a substantial role in the relatively poor longevity performance of the United States. (p. S-4)

> The damage caused by smoking was estimated to account for 78 percent of the gap in life expectancy for women and 41 percent of the gap for men between the United States and other high income countries in 2003. (p. S-2)

> Obesity may account for a fifth to a third of the shortfall of life expectancy in the United States relative to the other countries studied. (p. S-2)

What are the implications of these conclusions for future trends in life expectancy? Mortality will likely continue to decline as further progress is made in medicine, biotechnology, public health, nutrition, access to medical services, incomes, and education. However, substantial disagreement exists among analysts about how rapidly future improvements will occur (Bongaarts, 2006; Wilmoth, 1997 and 2001). At one end of the spectrum of opinion are pessimists (Carnes, Olshansky, and Grahn, 1996; Olshansky et al., 2005), who believe that the most advanced countries are close to a biological limit to longevity. A very different opinion is held by optimists (Oeppen and Vaupel, 2002), who expect life expectancy at birth to continue to rise very rapidly, reaching over 100 years later this century. Most projections by researchers and government agencies fall between these extremes (Lee and Carter, 1992; Li and Lee, 2005; Tuljapurkar, Li, and Boe, 2000; Bongaarts, 2006). The best-known U.S. projection is the one used by the Social Security Administration. The 2011 Report of the Board of Trustees of the Federal Old-Age and Survivors Insurance and Federal Disability Insurance Trust Funds (commonly known as the Trustees Report) projects life expectancy to reach 82.2 years in 2050, up from 77.7 in 2006.

In 2010 the Social Security Advisory Board appointed the Technical Panel on Assumptions and Methods (TPAM) to assess the assumptions and methods used in the Trustees Report. The TPAM made a number of recommendations, including a significant revision of mortality projections. The conclusion that increases in life expectancy will likely be more rapid than is currently assumed in the Trustees Report is based on an analysis of potential future trends in smoking and obesity (Technical Panel on Assumptions and Methods, 2011). The TPAM noted that the slow pace of improvement in life expectancy over recent decades was due to the impact of smoking and obesity and that these behavioral effects will likely continue to depress U.S. life expectancy. However, after rising for decades, indicators for smoking and obesity have now plateaued. According to the 2011 NRC report mentioned above:

> After 1964, when the Surgeon General's Office released its authoritative report on the adverse effects of cigarette smoking, the increase in smoking slowed, stopped and eventually reversed in the United States. (p. S-4)
>
> Recent data on obesity for the United States suggest that its prevalence has leveled off and some studies indicate that the mortality risk associated with obesity has declined. (p. S-4)

The TPAM therefore assumed that the adverse impact of these behaviors on life expectancy will remain at, or close to, current levels rather than rise much further in the future. Taking these trends into account, the TPAM expects U.S. life expectancy to reach 84.5 years in 2050. This estimate is close to a widely used and respected projection made by Li and Lee (2005) but above the 2011 Trustees Report assumption of 82.2 years. As shown in Figure 3-1, the future pace of improvement is more rapid than assumed in the Trustees Report but still slightly slower than the pace achieved by other high-income countries in past decades.

The projections of life expectancy, population aging, and other demographic indicators used in the present report are based on special projections made by the committee to incorporate the higher trend in life expectancy recommended by the Social Security TPAM (see Appendix A).

Life Expectancy at Older Ages

Remaining male life expectancy for those aged 65 in 2010 equaled 17.5 years, but it dropped to 10.8 years for those aged 75 and to 5.7 years at age 85 (Table 3-1). At all ages women have more years remaining than men. The committee's projections indicate an ongoing upward trend in remaining life expectancy at these older ages as well, with life expectancy at 65 reaching 22.2 years for males and 24.1 years for females in 2050. It is noteworthy that Japanese females had already achieved in 2009 the life expectancy that U.S. women are not projected to reach until 2050 (Organisation for Economic Co-operation and Development, 2011). The declines in remain-

TABLE 3-1 Years of Remaining Life at Older Ages in the United States: 1950, 2010, and 2050

Age	Gender	1950	2010	2050
65	Male	12.8	17.5	22.2
	Female	15.1	19.9	24.1
75	Male	7.9	10.8	14.2
	Female	9.0	12.5	15.6
85	Male	4.5	5.7	7.6
	Female	5.0	6.7	8.5

SOURCES: 1950 and 2010 from Board of Trustees, Federal Old-Age and Survivors Insurance and Federal Disability Insurance Trust Funds (2011); 2050 from special projections prepared by the committee (see Appendix A).

ing life expectancy as people age are important for the later discussion of public support systems such as Social Security and Medicare.

Longer Life and the Individual Life Cycle

As discussed later in this chapter, population aging results in part from longer life and in part from lower fertility. Figure 3-2 plots the average number of years spent in the three main life cycle phases: (1) total not working (during childhood or adult years prior to age 60); (2) working (defined as being in the labor force); and (3) retired (over age 60 and not in the labor force). The sum of the years spent in these three phases equals the life expectancy at birth, as plotted in Figure 3-1.[1]

As longevity rises over time, people spend more time in retirement. Between 1962 and 2010 the average time spent in retirement rose by 5 years (from 10 to 15 years), while life expectancy rose by 8 years. During this period, years in the labor force increased modestly but years not working declined slightly. These trends are largely attributable to the increasing labor force participation of women (see Chapter 5). In 1950, only 10.6 years were spent retired, but by 2050 the years in retirement are projected to reach 20, nearly doubling, while working years rise from 31 to 40 and nonworking years remain nearly constant.

The U.S. population is devoting increasing years to retirement both in absolute terms and as a proportion of life. As shown in Figure 3-3, the proportion of life spent in retirement rose from 15 to 19 percent between 1962 and 2010 and is expected to reach 24 percent in 2050. The ratio of retired

---

[1] Estimates are based on labor force participation rates by age through 2010 provided by the Office of Critical Trends Analysis of the Social Security Administration. Labor force participation rates are held constant from 2010 to 2050.

DEMOGRAPHIC TRENDS 37

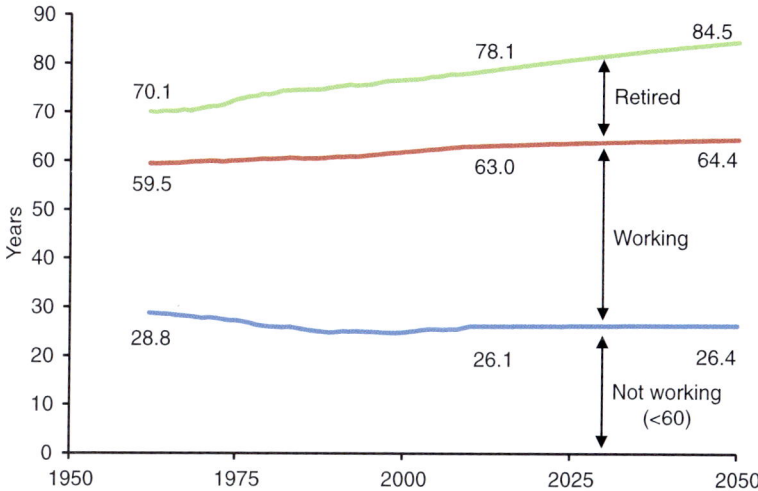

FIGURE 3-2 Years lived retired, working, and not working, 1962-2050. SOURCES: Board of Trustees, Federal Old-Age and Survivors Insurance and Federal Disability Insurance Trust Funds (2011) and projections by the committee.

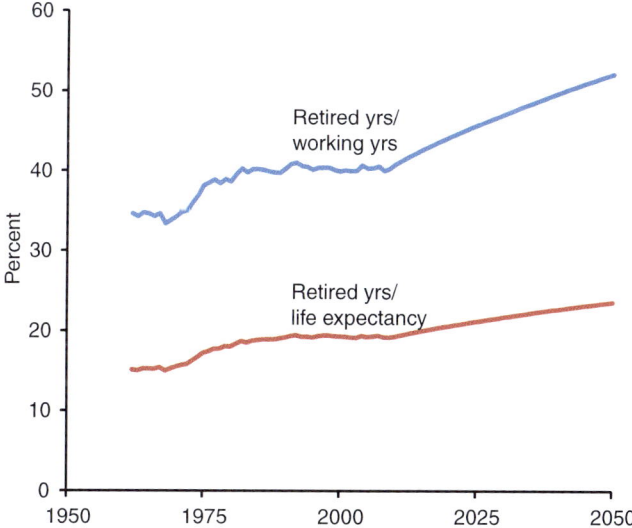

FIGURE 3-3 Retired years as a proportion of working years and of life expectancy, 1962-2050. SOURCES: Board of Trustees, Federal Old-Age and Survivors Insurance and Federal Disability Insurance Trust Funds (2011); and projections by the committee.

to working years also grew from 35 to 41 percent between 1962 and 2010. By 2050 this proportion is projected to be 52 percent, which implies that the average individual would then work 2 years for every year in retirement.

Adjusting the Life Cycle

As discussed in later chapters of this report, the costs of public support for health and pension benefits to the elderly will be difficult to bear given the rapid pace of population aging. Among the adaptations that are being considered is an increase in the age at retirement with full benefits, because the costs of this public support decline as the age of eligibility rises. It is useful to consider two simple demographic calculations to put this adaptation in context. In the first, we ask until what age a person would have to work in 2050 in order to have the same number of years in retirement as someone who retired at age 65 in 2010. The answer is 70.2 years.

Another useful calculation would be how many more years of work will be needed in the future to keep the ratio of retired years to working years constant at the 2010 level.[2] As shown in Figure 3-4, a retirement age of just 60 years would have yielded the same ratio in 1950 as in 2010. Based on the committee's projections, a rise of 4 years (from 65 to 69) would hold this ratio unchanged between 2010 and 2050. This scenario involves a smaller rise in the age at retirement and would allow some increase in years spent in retirement.

Socioeconomic and Geographic Variations in U.S. Life Expectancy

The preceding discussion focused on the average life expectancy in the United States and other countries. In addition to between-country variation in life expectancy there is substantial within-country variation, e.g., among racial and ethnic groups, among states and counties, and among groups with different levels of education and income.

Table 3-2 presents life expectancy for whites and blacks in 2008. White life expectancy at birth exceeds black life expectancy by 5 years (75.9 vs. 70.9) among males and by 3.4 years (80.8 vs. 77.4) among females. By age 65, these racial differences have declined to 1.8 years for males and 1.0 year for females. Analyses of ethnic differences usually find mortality among Hispanics to be lower than among whites. This so-called "Hispanic paradox" is probably due to a selection for good health among immigrants from Latin America and a tendency of Hispanic immigrants to return to their

---

[2]For this simulation, working years are calculated as years lived between age 20 and retirement age in a stationary population with current life expectancy. Retired years equal years of life remaining after retirement. Age at retirement is set at 65 in 2010.

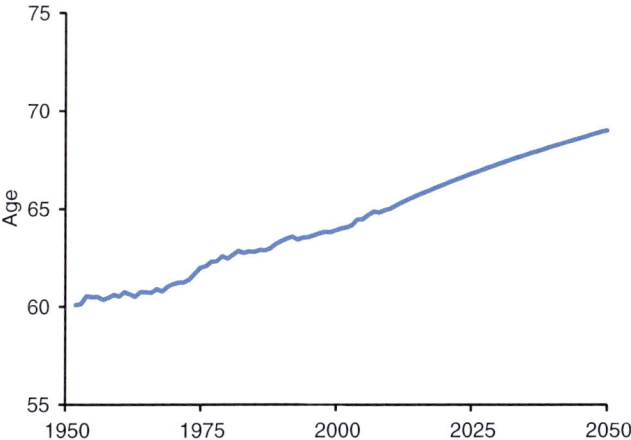

FIGURE 3-4 Hypothetical retirement age required to keep the 2010 ratio of retired to working years constant through 2050. SOURCES: Board of Trustees, Federal Old-Age and Survivors Insurance and Federal Disability Insurance Trust Funds (2011) and projections by the committee.

country of origin when they become ill (Elo and Preston, 1997; Markides and Eschbach, 2011).

Large mortality differences due to education level are found in the United States as well as in other countries. As shown in Table 3-3, life expectancy at age 25 in 1998 was 7.6 years less for males with less than 9 years of schooling compared to males with 13 or more years of schooling. Among females the difference between these two groups was 4.9 years. At age 65 these differences narrowed but remained a substantial 3.4 years for males and 2.5 years for females. A more recent analysis of trends through 2008 found that adults with fewer than 12 years of education in 2008 had life expectancies similar to the U.S. average in the 1950s and 1960s

TABLE 3-2 Years of Life Expectancy at Birth and at Age 65 for Whites and Blacks, 2008

	White	Black	Difference (White − Black)
At birth	78.4	74.3	4.1
Male	75.9	70.9	5.0
Female	80.8	77.4	3.4
At age 65	18.7	17.5	1.2
Male	17.3	15.5	1.8
Female	19.9	18.9	1.0

SOURCE: U.S. Census Bureau (2012).

TABLE 3-3 Years of Life Expectancy at Ages 25 and 65 by Educational Attainment, 1998

	Years of Schooling			
	0-8	9-12	13+	Difference (13+) − (0-8)
At age 25				
Male	47.0	47.5	54.6	7.6
Female	52.9	53.6	57.8	4.9
At age 65				
Male	14.9	15.1	18.3	3.4
Female	17.9	18.3	20.4	2.5

SOURCES: Data from Hummer and Lariscy (2011); Molla, Madans, and Wagener (2004).

(Olshansky et al., 2012). By combining education and race, the study showed large and growing differences in life expectancy between whites with 16+ years of schooling compared to blacks with fewer than 12 years of education.

Geographic differences in mortality are also well established. Life expectancy in 1999-2001 was highest in Hawaii and Minnesota and lowest in the District of Columbia and Mississippi (Table 3-4). Differences at the county level are even larger than among states (Ezzati et al., 2008).

The literature has proposed a range of factors that may be responsible for or contribute to these mortality differences. Generally, disadvantaged groups or populations smoke more, are more obese, exercise less, live more stressful lives; have less access to health care services; have fewer social resources and lower status occupations; live in neighborhoods with poor housing, high levels of pollution, and relatively high crime rates; and have less income and education (Centers for Disease Control and Prevention, 2011; National Research Council, 2004a, 2004b). Differences in genetic endowment may also play a role (Christensen and Vaupel, 2011). Despite the often significant correlation between these explanatory factors and mortality, it is difficult to disentangle the complex causal pathways and quantify the true determinants of mortality differences.

TABLE 3-4 Years of Life Expectancy at Birth and at Age 50 for Selected States/Areas, 1991-2001

	District of Columbia	Mississippi	.....	Minnesota	Hawaii	Difference (Hawaii − D.C.)
At birth	72.3	73.6		79.0	79.7	7.4
At age 50	28.0	31.4		31.4	32.4	4.4

SOURCE: Wilmoth, Boe, and Barbieri (2010).

These mortality differences have potentially important implications for the design of policies to address the adverse consequences of aging. In particular, raising the full retirement age for all retirees leads to a larger proportional reduction in expected years of retired life for disadvantaged groups than for advantaged groups. The committee believes that such a differential impact would be undesirable.

POPULATION AGING

Population Age Distribution

The older population in the United States is on the threshold of a boom. The population aged 65 and over will increase substantially between 2010 and 2030, reaching 72 million in 2030, more than twice the level (35 million) in the year 2000 (He et al., 2005; Vincent and Velkoff, 2010). Figure 3-5 shows broad changes in the nation's age distribution from 1950 to 2010 and projected changes through 2050. This graphic highlights the growing share of people in older age groups and the corresponding decline in the share of the population under age 30. As discussed in more depth later in this chapter, the United States is aging less rapidly than most other high-income countries and may be relatively better able to cope with the pressures of demographic change.

Another view of changing age distribution is provided by Figure 3-6, which plots U.S. population size by age for 1975 and 2000 and as projected to 2025 and 2050. In 1975 a large proportion of the population was between 10 and 30 years of age. This group is often referred to as the baby boom generation, because it consists of the survivors of the large number of U.S. births between 1945 and 1965. As this generation ages, its presence in the age structure leaves a visible bulge that reaches ages 35-55 in 2000, ages 60-80 in 2025, and ages 85+ in 2050. The population aged 90+ rises more than 17-fold between 1975 and 2050. Over past decades, the baby boom postponed population aging as it moved through the labor force ages. But now it is ushering in a new period of very rapid population aging as it moves into old age.

The baby boom generation retires during the first quarter of the twenty-first century, causing a steep increase in the number of recipients of Social Security and Medicare benefits (Figure 3-7). The number of people reaching age 65 each year rose modestly between 1950 and 1980 and then fell for several years as a result of low birth rates during the Depression years of the 1930s. But between 2000 and 2025 the annual number of those turning age 65 is expected to more than double, from 2.1 to 4.3 million (the modest reduction after 2025 is due to the end of the baby boom in the 1960s).

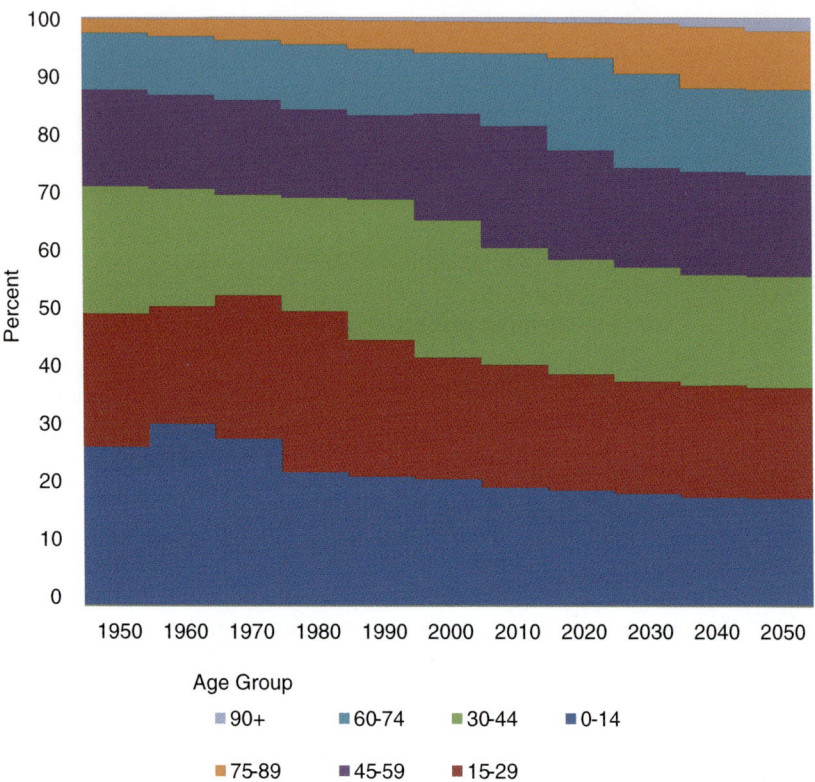

FIGURE 3-5 Percent distribution of the population by age, 1950-2050. SOURCES: Board of Trustees, Federal Old-Age and Survivors Insurance and Federal Disability Insurance Trust Funds (2011) and projections by the committee.

Providing pensions and health care for this wave of new retirees will be a challenge.

Demographic Drivers of Aging

The amount of aging the U.S. population will experience in the future depends on trends in mortality, fertility, and migration. In general, the lower the levels of fertility, mortality, and migration, the older the population will become. It should be stressed that if infant and younger-adult mortality rates remain relatively low for a prolonged time, as has been the case in most developed countries for many decades, changes in life expectancy at older ages become inceasingly important to changes in overall life expectancy. The demographic assumptions on fertility, mortality, and migration underlying the population projections in this report are discussed next.

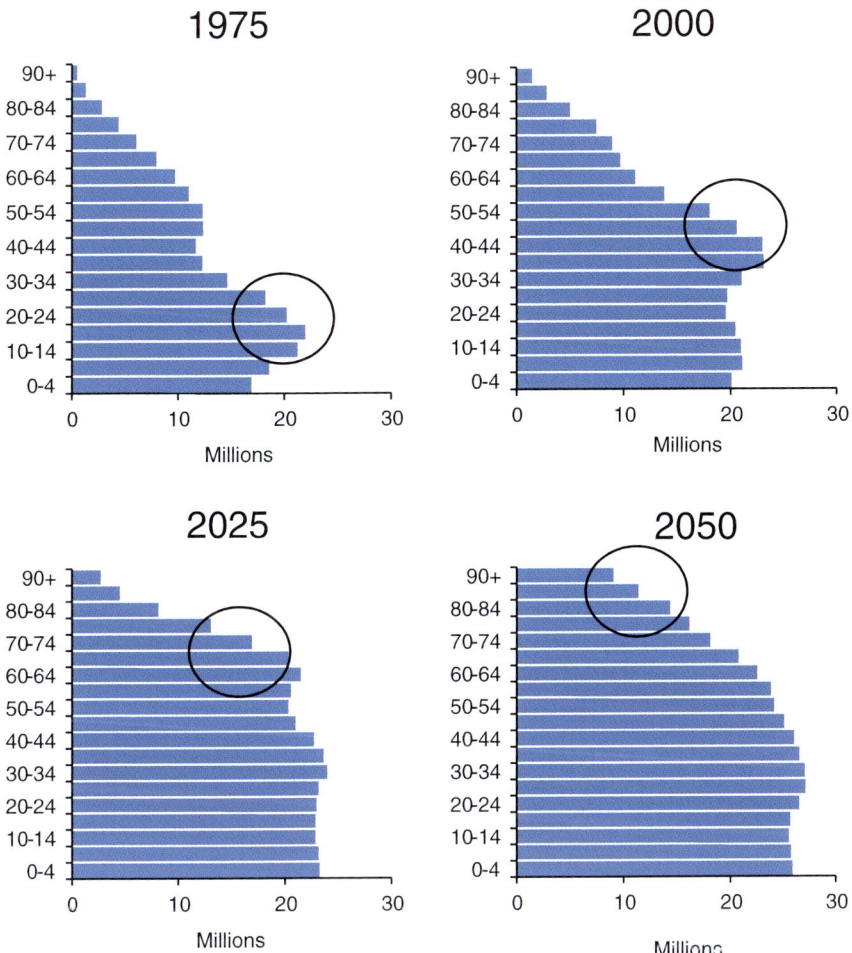

FIGURE 3-6 Population by age, 1975-2050. The circled groups approximate the baby boom as it moves through time. SOURCES: Board of Trustees, Federal Old-Age and Survivors Insurance and Federal Disability Insurance Trust Funds (2011) and projections by the committee.

Fertility

Past estimates and projections of fertility as measured by the total fertility rate (TFR) are plotted in Figure 3-8. Over the past half-century the TFR has fluctuated widely in response to a range of social and economic developments. Fertility rose sharply after the Second World War, reaching 3.7 births per woman at the peak of the baby boom in 1957. The next two

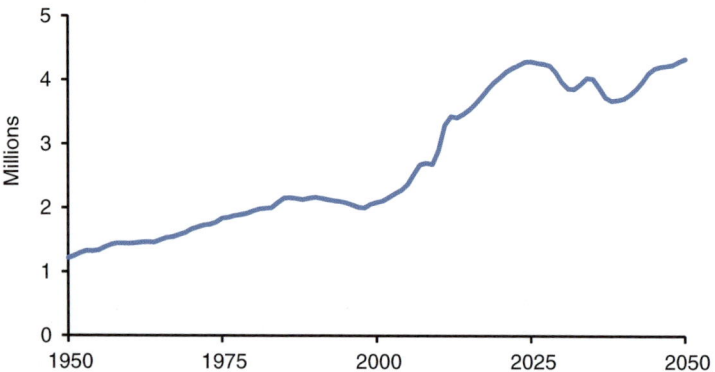

FIGURE 3-7 Number of people turning 65, 1950-2050. SOURCES: Board of Trustees, Federal Old-Age and Survivors Insurance and Federal Disability Insurance Trust Funds (2011) and projections by the committee.

decades saw a steep decline to 1.7 births per woman in 1976. Over the next three decades, the TFR slowly recovered, reaching an average just below 2.1 during the period 2006-2010.[3] The 2011 Trustees Report assumes a small decline to 2.0 will occur over the next two decades. This assumption was reviewed by the 2011 TPAM and found to be reasonable, and it is incorporated into the population projections used in this report.

Mortality

As noted earlier, the Social Security Advisory Board's TPAM has recommended assuming a U.S. life expectancy of 84.5 years in 2050, and this assumption has been adopted in the population projections used in the present report.

Migration

Net migration, legal and illegal, rose from 0.8 to 1.9 million per year between 1980 and 2005 (see Figure 3-9, solid line). The recession of the late 2000s reduced this number to near zero in 2008, followed by a rebound in 2009 and 2010. These large recent swings are mostly due to changes in illegal migration, which is estimated to have turned negative in 2007. Legal

---

[3]The total fertility rate was between 2.0 and 2.1 births per woman during the period 2000-2005 and reached 2.1 in 2006 and 2007. The TFR declined modestly after 2007 in conjunction with the economic downturn, to a level between 1.9 and 2.0 according to preliminary 2010 data (National Center for Health Statistics, 2011).

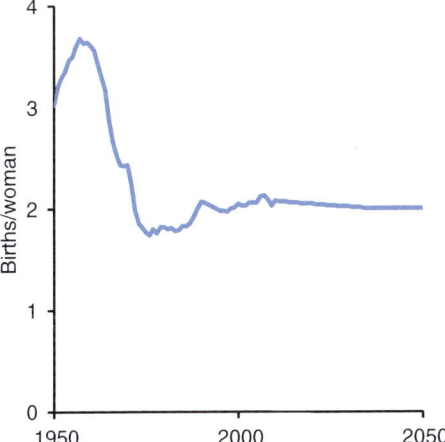

FIGURE 3-8 Total fertility rate, 1950-2050. SOURCE: Board of Trustees, Federal Old-Age and Survivors Insurance and Federal Disability Insurance Trust Funds (2011).

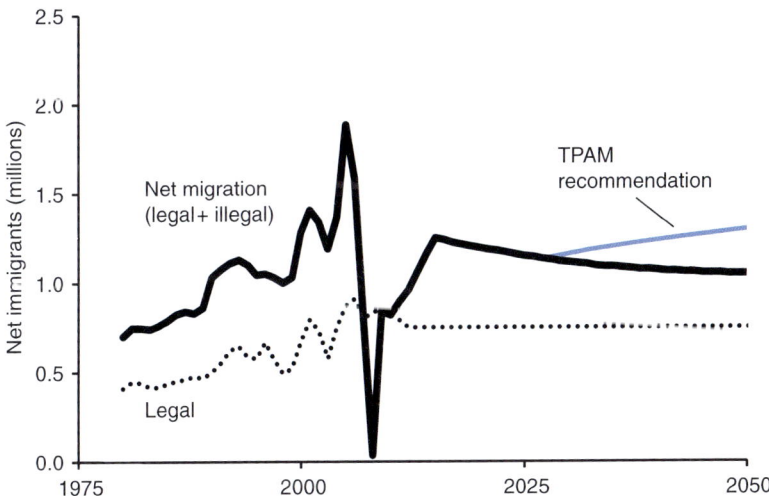

FIGURE 3-9 Net migration, 1980-2050. SOURCES: Board of Trustees, Federal Old-Age and Survivors Insurance and Federal Disability Insurance Trust Funds (2011) and Technical Panel on Assumptions and Methods (2011).

net migration shows only minor fluctuations. The fairly steady past rise in legal migration comes from the implementation of new legislation allowing a larger influx in recent decades.

The Social Security Trustees Report projects that the rebound in migration will continue until 2015 before beginning a steady decline over future decades. This decline is assumed to be entirely in illegal migration; legal migration is held constant at 750,000 from 2012 onward following current law. The TPAM reviewed these projections and accepted the projections from 2010 to 2025 but recommended an increase in the projected flow of migrants after 2025. There are two main reasons for this recommendation: (1) the population of the United States and the sending countries is expected to grow in future decades and (2) current law will probably change to allow more legal migration. The projections in the present report incorporate this higher migration trajectory recommended by the TPAM.

Because migrants are on average younger than the U.S. population, migration reduces population aging. The impact of migration can be es-

---

BOX 3-1
The Impact of Demographic Alternatives

Since trends in fertility, migration, and mortality are the direct determinants of trends in the population age structure, it is reasonable to consider policies that could reduce future population aging by changing these determinants. Raising mortality is, of course, not a realistic option, but fertility and migration could be changed through government intervention.

To illustrate the likely effects of demographic alternatives, the committee poses the question, How would levels of fertility and migration have to change (relative to the committee's preferred assumptions—see Appendix A) to achieve a 10 percent reduction in the old age dependency ratio (OADR) by the year 2050? In other words, what amount of change would reduce the expected 2050 OADR of about 0.39 shown in Figure 3-13 to 0.35?

Current projections made by the Social Security Trustees and accepted by the committee assume that the U.S. total fertility rate will decline very modestly from about 2.1 births per woman during the period 2006-2010 to 2.0 births by 2035 and remain constant until 2050. In order to achieve a 10 percent reduction in the projected OADR, the total fertility rate would have to increase by 0.5 birth per woman between now and 2035 and then remain constant (assuming no concurrent change in mortality or migration). Thus, an OADR of 0.35 in 2050 would require a 25 percent increase in the total fertility rate, from 2.0 to 2.5.

Higher fertility would reduce population aging but at the same time raise the population growth rate and lead to a larger future population. Hence, there is a trade-off between the gains from a younger population and the costs of a larger population, including environmental costs. And it is unclear what might prompt such a rise in fertil-

timated by comparing the standard projection (which includes migration) with a hypothetical projection in which migration is set to zero from 2010 onwards. The former expects the proportion of the population aged 65+ to reach 21 percent in 2050, while the latter expects a substantially higher 24 percent. In contrast, if the migration rate is projected to be twice the rate in the standard projection, the proportion of the population aged 65+ declines to 19 percent. These estimates of the impact of changes in future migration are probably somewhat conservative because they ignore secondary effects on fertility and mortality, which are difficult to assess (see Box 3-1 for an alternative illustration of the impact of migration).

The projections presented in this report differ from those made in the Trustees Report because the committee has adopted the TPAM assumptions regarding future trends in mortality and migration. According to the actuaries of the Social Security Administration, the change in the mortality assumption raises the deficit in the system balance in 2060 from −3.55 percent to −4.33 percent while the change in the migration assumption

---

ity. Pronatalist financial incentives have had relatively little effect on fertility when they have been tried in other countries, particularly in Europe. It is easier to alter the timing of a woman's fertility than it is to alter the eventual number of children that she has (Hoorens et al., 2011; Kohler, Billari, and Ortega, 2006).

Higher net immigration, both documented and undocumented, would also reduce population aging, but like higher fertility, would lead to faster population growth and larger size. Because immigrants themselves become old, the long-term effect of immigration on population aging is less than might be expected (United Nations, 2001). In the example here, a 10 percent reduction in the OADR by 2050 would require an average annual increase of 69 percent in the rate of net immigration during the period 2010-2050. In absolute terms, this would mean an average of nearly 1 million more net immigrants each year.

In the past, immigrants had substantially higher fertility than the native population, although not as much higher as was often thought (Parrado, 2011). But fertility has fallen rapidly in many of the source countries—for example, to around 1.6 births per woman in China and 2.3 births per woman in Mexico—so the effects of immigration on fertility in the United States will most likely be smaller than before. Again, there is a trade-off between reduced population aging and increased population size, and there are well-known controversies surrounding levels of immigration. The economic, social, and demographic consequences of immigration were analyzed in earlier National Research Council reports (1997; 2001).

The conventional OADR is calculated as the ratio of population over 64 ("old dependents") to the population aged 20-64 ("working age"). Age 65 is the boundary between these groups and represents the assumed retirement age. A reduction in the OADR can therefore also be achieved by raising this age boundary. In fact, a rise in this age from 65.0 to 66.7 would produce a decline of 10 percent in the OADR in 2050.

reduces this deficit from −3.55 percent to −3.36 percent (Technical Panel on Assumptions and Methods, 2011). The mortality change is clearly much more consequential than the migration change.

WHY POPULATION AGING MATTERS: AGE PATTERNS OF CONSUMPTION AND LABOR INCOME

Population aging matters because average economic behavior varies systematically with age. It is interesting to estimate how consumption and labor income have actually varied across age at different periods over the past half century. Such estimates are shown in Figures 3-10 and 3-11 for 1960, 1981, and 2007. Consumption includes private household expenditures that are imputed to the members of each household in proportion to an assumed set of age-weights. It also includes in-kind public transfers to individuals of public education and of publicly provided health care through Medicare and Medicaid, including long-term care. Labor income includes wages and salaries and fringe benefits, plus two-thirds of self-employment income (the other third is counted as a return to property or assets such as a farm or family store). To make these "age profiles" easier to compare across calendar years, they are divided by the average level of labor income between ages 30 and 49 in each calendar year.

Figure 3-10 shows several important changes over the half-century. At younger ages, there was a large increase in expenditures on public education and an accompanying increase in private spending for college education. Most interesting here, however, are the changes in adulthood, particularly at older ages. In 1960 total consumption declined substantially after age 60

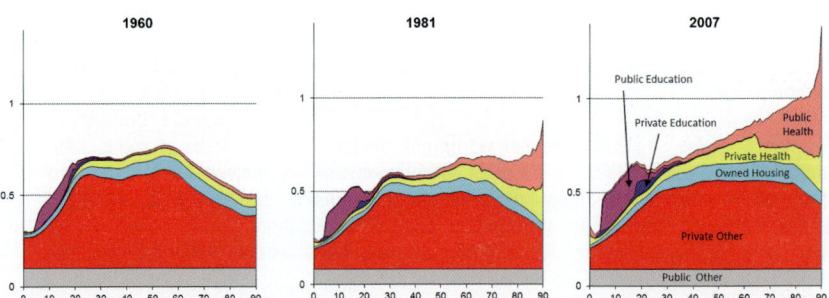

FIGURE 3-10 The age profile of U.S. consumption, 1960, 1981, and 2007. For each year, all values have been divided by average labor income in that year between ages 30-49 to standardize for visual comparison of shapes. SOURCE: Special tabulations by Lee and Donehower using data from the National Transfer Accounts project; see Lee and Mason (2011, Chapter 9) for details and methods.

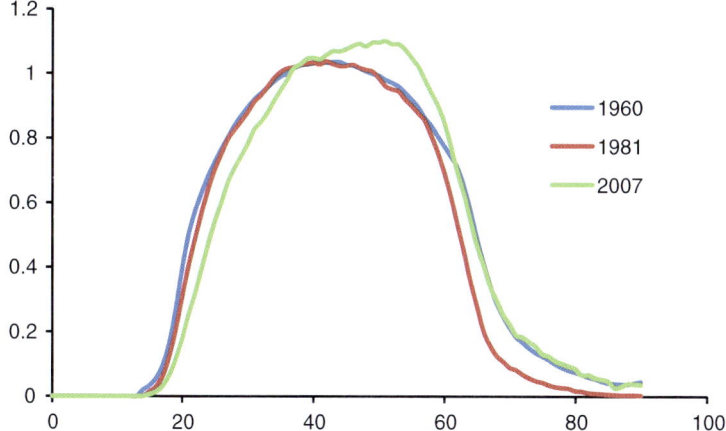

FIGURE 3-11 U.S. labor income by age, 1960, 1981, and 2007. Labor income is before taxes and includes fringe benefits and two-thirds of self-employment income. For each year, all values have been divided by average labor income in that year between ages 30 and 49. SOURCE: Special tabulations by Lee and Donehower using data from the National Transfer Accounts project; see Lee and Mason (2011, Chapter 9) for details and methods.

owing to the decline in "Private Other" spending—that is, all household consumption other than health, education, and services from owned housing. This predated Medicare and Medicaid, and public expenditures on health care were no greater for elderly individuals than for younger adults. By 1981, "Private Other" consumption did not begin to decline until age 70. Private spending on health rose substantially with age, and public spending on health care rose even more strongly with age. Total consumption rose across adult ages in 1981 in contrast to its decline in 1960, and rose strongly after age 85.

By 2007 these changes had intensified. Private nonhealth consumption did not decline until age 80 in 2007 as compared with age 70 in 1981 and age 60 in 1960. Most striking was the expansion of public spending on health care. We also see a sharp reduction in private spending on health care at age 65 and a corresponding increase in public spending through Medicare. Total consumption is now seen to rise strongly with age. In 1960 an 80-year-old consumed 83 percent of what a 20-year-old consumed. By 1981 an 80-year-old consumed 39 percent more than a 20-year-old, and by 2007 an 80-year-old consumed 67 percent more. The ratio of consumption at age 80 to age 20 doubled since 1960.

Comparable estimates are available for labor income (Figure 3-11). In 1960 and 1981, the labor income curve for the 20s and early 30s is shifted

3 to 4 years toward younger age relative to the curve for 2007. The 1960 and 1981 curves are virtually identical until age 60. After age 60, the 1960 curve is virtually coincident with the 2007 curve and is shifted 2 to 3 years toward older ages relative to 1981. In the 70s age range it is shifted many years toward older ages.[4]

The result of these changes in the economic life cycle is that consumption in old age net of labor income has become much more costly. Population aging will occur rapidly over the coming decades as the baby boom moves into older ages, and the societal costs will be heightened by the corresponding increase in the net consumption of the elderly. At the same time, the elderly in the United States continue to earn a substantial amount of labor income, more than in most other industrial nations (Lee and Mason, 2011).

INDICATORS OF POPULATION AGING AND ITS ECONOMIC IMPACT

Demographers and economists use a range of indicators to compare the degree of population aging over time and between countries. The most basic of these measures can be calculated for all countries but have shortcomings that limit their usefulness; the more complex ones require more detailed data but are better suited to analyses of the economic impact of aging. One key point is that the correspondence between chronological age on the one hand and health and vitality on the other has changed dramatically in recent decades, as reflected in the popular saying "70 is the new 60." These changes will be discussed in the next chapter, and must be kept in mind even as "the elderly" continue to be defined as people aged 65 and over.

Proportion of Population Aged 65 and Over

In 2010, 13 percent of the U.S. population was over the age of 64, up from 8 percent in 1950. This proportion is expected to jump above 20 percent over the next two decades as the baby boom generation retires, before plateauing in the 2030s and 2040s (Figure 3-12). The proportions aged 75+ and 85+ follow a similar path but at a lower level. Moreover, the upswings occur later, with a delay of 10 years for the 75+ population and 20 years for the 85+ population.

---

[4]Throughout this discussion of consumption and labor income we are comparing values across ages in the same time period. Actual paths of earning and consuming over the lifetime of a generation would have different shapes, tilted upwards and shifted to older ages, because productivity growth leads to growing income and consumption as generations move through their lives.

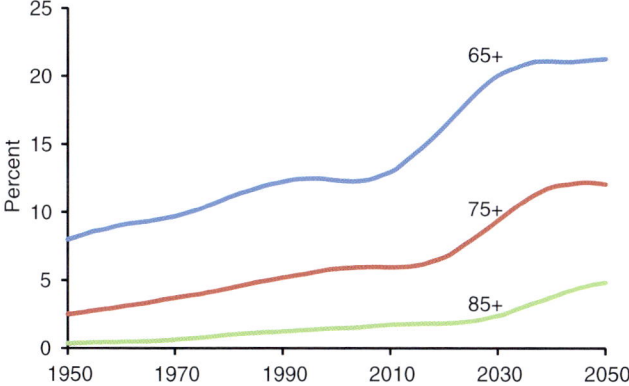

FIGURE 3-12 Share of population aged 65+, 75+, and 85+, 1950-2050. SOURCES: Board of Trustees, Federal Old-Age and Survivors Insurance and Federal Disability Insurance Trust Funds (2011) and projections by the committee.

Age Dependency Ratio

The age dependency ratio (ADR) is the ratio of population aged 65 and over plus those under 20 ("dependents") to the working age population (ages 20-64). Figure 3-13 plots estimates of the ADR for the United States from 1950 to 2010 and projections to 2050. The ADR fluctuates substantially over time but shows no clear long-range trend. It reached its

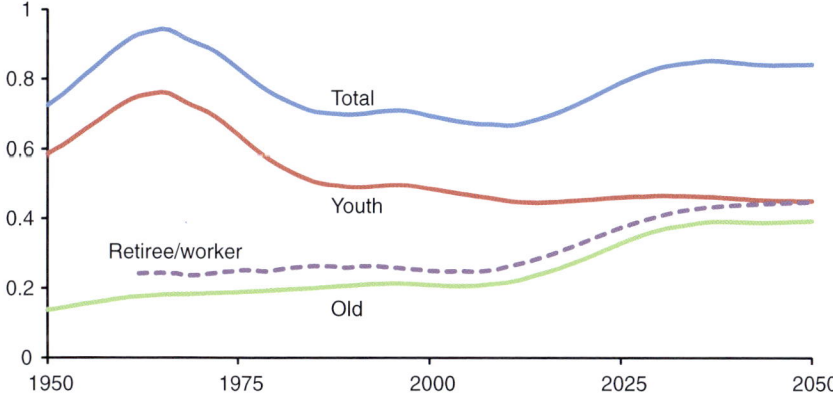

FIGURE 3-13 Age dependency ratios, 1950-2050. SOURCES: Board of Trustees, Federal Old-Age and Survivors Insurance and Federal Disability Insurance Trust Funds (2011) and projections by the committee.

peak value, 0.94, in 1965 then declined to its minimum, 0.67, in 2010 and is projected to rise again to a new peak, 0.85, in 2037.

To explain this trend it is useful to examine the two components of the ADR: the old age dependency ratio (OADR, population 65+/population 20-64) and the young age dependency ratio (YADR, population <20/population 20-64). As seen in Figure 3-13, these two components show very different trajectories over time. The YADR peak in 1965 was responsible for the first peak in the ADR, and the future rise in the OADR is responsible for the projected second peak in the ADR in the 2030s. As a result of these opposing trends in the OADR and YADR, the composition of dependents shifts from mostly under age 20 in the 1960s to nearly even between old and young dependents in 2050.

Although widely used, this ratio has a key flaw: It implicitly assumes that all people aged under 20 and over 64 are "dependents" and that all people aged 20-64 are "working." These assumptions are at best an approximation of reality, and the quality of this approximation changes over time both because of changes in actual economic behavior and because of changes in underlying health.

Retiree to Worker Ratio

The retiree/worker ratio (RWR) can be considered an improved version of the old age dependency ratio. The numerator of the RWR consists of the number of retirees (instead of the population 65+) and its denominator consists of all people in the labor force (instead of the population aged 20-64). The RWR typically exceeds the OADR by a small amount because the number of retirees exceeds the population aged 65+ and because the number of workers is somewhat smaller than the population aged 20-64. The trends over time in the two indicators are similar, as shown in Figure 3-13, where the dashed line represents the RWR.

Support Ratio

Unweighted

Support ratios differ from dependency ratios in that the supporters (or workers) are in the numerator and the dependents (or consumers) are in the denominator; these measures are therefore inversely related to dependency ratios. The simplest support ratio is the proportion of the population that is working. The numerator consists of everyone in the labor force[5] and the denominator equals the entire population, all of whom are consumers. The

---

[5] "Labor force" is defined in Chapter 5.

DEMOGRAPHIC TRENDS

unweighted support ratio (SRU) rose from 1962 to 1980 then plateaued until 2010, but it is expected to decline by 2050 (Figure 3-14). The disadvantage of this measure is that it assumes that workers of all ages have equal incomes and that the same amount is consumed by people of all ages.

Weighted

The weighted support ratio (SRW) is a more sophisticated measure that improves on the unweighted version by allowing incomes of workers and consumption levels to vary by age. Specifically, the age patterns of consumption and labor income discussed previously (see Figure 3-10) are applied to the population by age to calculate the SRW. The ratio depends on the base year age profiles of consumption and labor income that are used. These are held constant to isolate the effect of changing population age distributions. It is a hypothetical "other things equal" calculation, not an attempt to project what the future ratios of labor income to consumption will be.

Trends and projections of SRW are presented in Figure 3-14 (top line), based on the labor income and consumption profiles of 2007 combined with each year's population age distribution. The SRW is higher than the SRU mainly because income substantially exceeds consumption among

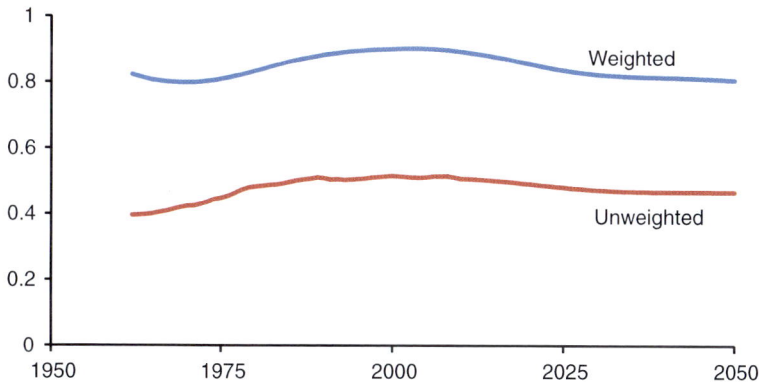

FIGURE 3-14 Unweighted and weighted support ratios, 1962-2050. SOURCES: Board of Trustees, Federal Old-Age and Survivors Insurance and Federal Disability Insurance Trust Funds (2011); Lee and Mason, 2011; and projections by the committee.

workers.[6] However the pattern of change in the SRW over time is similar to that of the SRU.

Table 3-5 summarizes estimates of six indicators in 2010 and 2050. These aging indicators differ because they are differently defined. Their absolute levels will not be examined here because there is little to be gained from a discussion of the differences. Instead the committee focuses on the projected trends (last column), which anticipate the future impact of population aging.

These results lead to two main conclusions regarding trends to 2050. First, the U.S. population will likely age substantially, as indicated by the 64 percent rise in the population aged 65+, the 81 percent rise in the OADR, and the 71 percent rise in the RWR. Second, the economic impact of this aging is cushioned by a decline in youth dependency.

The net effect of these demographic trends is best captured by the SRW, which is projected to decline 12 percent by 2050. This means that, other things being equal, consumption per capita will be 12 percent lower than it would be without population aging.[7]

Adapting to Population Aging

As noted throughout this report, adapting to future population aging might involve a rise in the age at retirement. Such an increase would counteract the projected adverse changes in most of the above indicators. To illustrate, Figure 3-15 plots the age at retirement (conventionally set at age 65) required to keep the OADR constant at 0.22. This calculation indicates that the age at retirement would have to rise from 65.0 in 2010 to 73.3 years in 2050 to prevent the OADR from increasing. A separate calculation indicates that a similar increase in age at retirement will keep the SRW constant. It should be emphasized that Figure 3-15 represents a purely hypothetical exercise to illustrate the magnitude of changes in age at retirement needed to keep this dependency ratio unchanged. Such a large change in age at retirement is likely to be politically unacceptable, and it is not the committee's intention to recommend it.

It is worth noting that this increase in the age at retirement of 8.3 years is larger than the rise of 4.0 years needed to keep the ratio of retired to working years constant over the individual life cycle (see earlier discussion of Figure 3-4). The reason for this difference is that the rise in the age at retirement plotted in Figure 3-15 compensates both for the projected rise in life expectancy and for population aging resulting from fertility decline

---

[6]The support ratio is typically less than unity because consumption is funded in part from sources other than labor income, such as asset income.

[7]That is, consumption per weighted consumer will decline by 12 percent, other things equal.

TABLE 3-5 Summary Indicators of Population Aging, 2010 and 2050

Indicator	2010	2050	Percent Change, 2010-2050
Aged 65+ (%)	13.0	21.3	64
ADR	.67	.84	26
OADR	.22	.39	81
RWR	.26	.45	71
SRU	.51	.47	−8
SRW	.78	.68	−12

SOURCES: Board of Trustees, Federal Old-Age and Survivors Insurance and Federal Disability Insurance Trust Funds (2011) and projections by the Committee.

and migration changes. In contrast, the life cycle calculations summarized in Figure 3-4 compensate only for rising life expectancy.

GLOBAL PATTERNS OF AGING

Population aging is occurring in most countries because life expectancy has risen and fertility has declined. Aging is most pronounced in high-income countries (i.e., Europe, North America, and Japan), where the median age of the population rose from 29 to 39 years between 1950 and 2010 (United Nations, 2011). United Nations projections expect this median to reach 48 years in 2050. Populations in the developing world (Asia excluding Japan, Latin America, and Africa) are generally younger, with

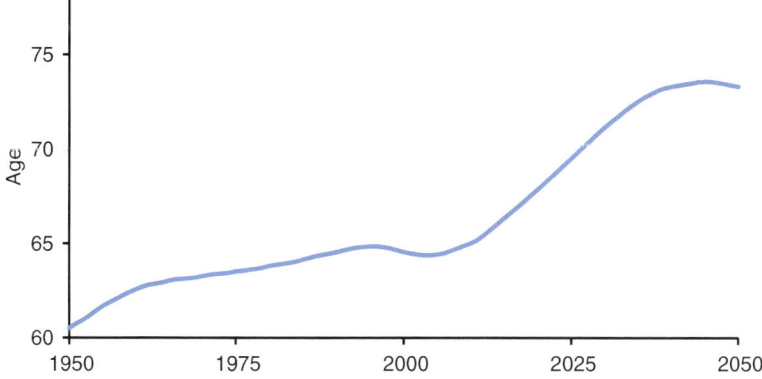

FIGURE 3-15 Retirement age required to keep old-age dependency ratio constant at its 2010 level. SOURCES: Board of Trustees, Federal Old-Age and Survivors Insurance and Federal Disability Insurance Trust Funds (2011) and projections by the committee.

a current aggregate median age of 27 years, but aging is also proceeding rapidly and the median is projected to reach 37 years in 2050.

Figure 3-16 plots past estimates and projections of the proportion aged 65+ for each of the world regions. Large regional differences are apparent. In 2010, proportions 65+ in Europe (16.2) and North America (13.2) are substantially higher than in Latin America (6.9), Asia (6.7) and Africa (3.5). By 2050 these proportions are expected to have risen further, reaching 26.9 percent in Europe and 21.6 percent in North America. The steepest increases are projected for Asia and Latin America, where levels will more than double and reach above today's European levels. Africa will also age, but slowly, and will remain the youngest region.

Figure 3-17 compares the United States with other high-income countries. By mid-century the proportion aged 65+ is projected to reach 21 percent in the United States and substantially higher in other rich countries (over 30 percent in Germany, Italy, and Spain and 36 percent in Japan). The reason for this difference is the relatively high fertility in the United States and the low fertility in Germany, Italy, Japan, and Spain. In addition, the United States is expected to have higher mortality and migration rates. Other high-income countries therefore face more pronounced aging than does the United States.

UNCERTAINTY IN POPULATION PROJECTIONS

It is obvious that many assumptions are required for a population projection. Painful actions such as raising the retirement age might be taken

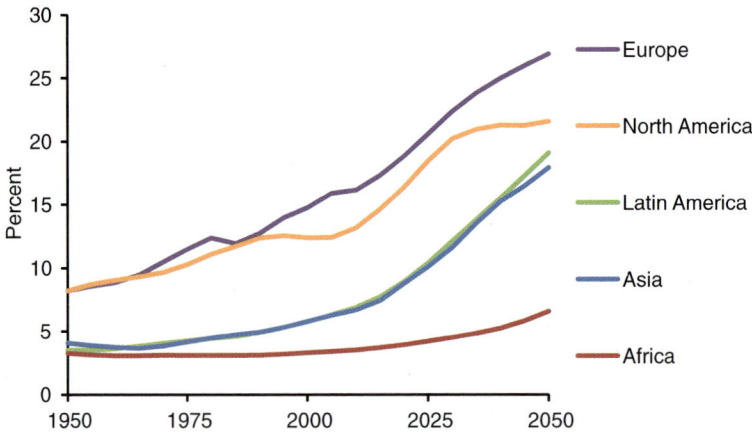

FIGURE 3-16 Share of the population aged 65+ in five world regions, 1950-2050.
SOURCE: United Nations (2011).

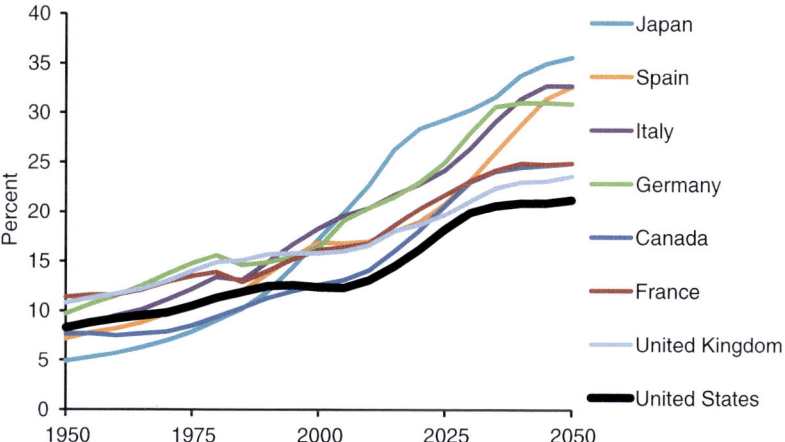

FIGURE 3-17 Share of population aged 65+ in eight high-income countries, 1950-2050. SOURCE: United Nations (2011).

now to ameliorate the consequences of projected population change far in the future. How certain can we be that the projected changes will actually occur and that action is needed now? To answer this important question, we need an indication of the uncertainty in the projections.

Demographers and statisticians have mainly used four different methods to assess the uncertainty of population projections (see National Research Council, 2000, for a detailed examination of both the accuracy of past projections and the uncertainty of population forecasts). The traditional method, which can be called "scenarios," is familiar to all: The projections are made in high, medium, and low variants, based on expert opinion about how high or low each of the key inputs—fertility, mortality, and net immigration—might be. This is certainly helpful, but there are difficulties with this approach. It seems to assume that if fertility (for example) is higher than expected in the first year of the projection, then it will also be higher in every subsequent year, and this assumption rules out the kinds of fluctuations that have occurred in the past. Because of this, the scenario method invites us to believe that if we just wait for a few years it will become clear whether the population is evolving according to the high or the low scenario, and uncertainty will be reduced. But this interpretation is mistaken. After a few years, a new set of scenarios would again feature similar high, medium, and low variants.

Construction of the scenarios also requires deciding whether to combine the high fertility assumption with a low mortality assumption or a high mortality assumption, and likewise for migration assumptions. This decision is essentially arbitrary, and however it is done, inconsistencies in the high-low ranges will result (see Lee, 1999).[8]

A second approach, called ex post analysis, analyzes the past record of success of forecasts prepared by an agency as a guide to the uncertainty of future forecasts. If the forecasting method has not changed too much over time, this method can be very useful. An unusually careful ex post analysis of the United Nations projections was provided by the National Research Council (2000).

A third approach might be called "random scenarios." It assumes a certain probability distribution of the true outcome in relation to high and low bounds provided by experts. Given this distribution, a process like the one described above can be used to generate possible future paths for each vital rate (Lutz, Sanderson, and Scherbov, 2004; Tuljapurkar, Li, and Boe, 2000).

A fourth approach is based on time-series analysis, which combines demographic methods with well-established statistical methods to model, analyze, and forecast historical data on fertility, mortality or migration (Lee and Tuljapurkar, 1994). The models capture not only the trend but also the typical patterns and degree of persistence of fluctuations. One can draw random numbers that, combined with the models, generate one possible version of the future of a particular rate—say fertility—that is consistent with the typical past patterns (Lee, 1999; 2011). In the same way, possible futures can be generated for mortality and net immigration. Then this set of randomly generated fertility, mortality, and migration outcomes can be used to generate a possible future trajectory for the population and its age distribution, say up to 2050. By repeating this process with a new set of random numbers, another possible future is generated. After 1,000 such repetitions, it becomes clear which outcomes are most likely and which are less likely, and it is possible to derive a probability distribution. This method produces not only a probability distribution of outcomes for a given year, but also a distribution of trajectories. Such an approach is valuable because some outcomes of interest, such as the projected Trust Fund balance for Social Security in a given year, depend not only on the demography of that particular year but also on the whole demographic trajectory leading up to that point, with all its ups and downs. In fact, the Social Security Trustees have included in their annual reports a stochastic forecast of this sort for the system's finances.

Figure 3-18 shows a probabilistic forecast of the OADR based on a stochastic version of the committee's single-sex population projection, for

---

[8]In effect, the scenario method assumes that projection errors in each component are perfectly correlated over time (always too high or always too low), and that errors in the different components are always perfectly positively or negatively correlated with one another (if fertility is high, then mortality or immigration is low, for example). Neither assumption is correct.

DEMOGRAPHIC TRENDS   59

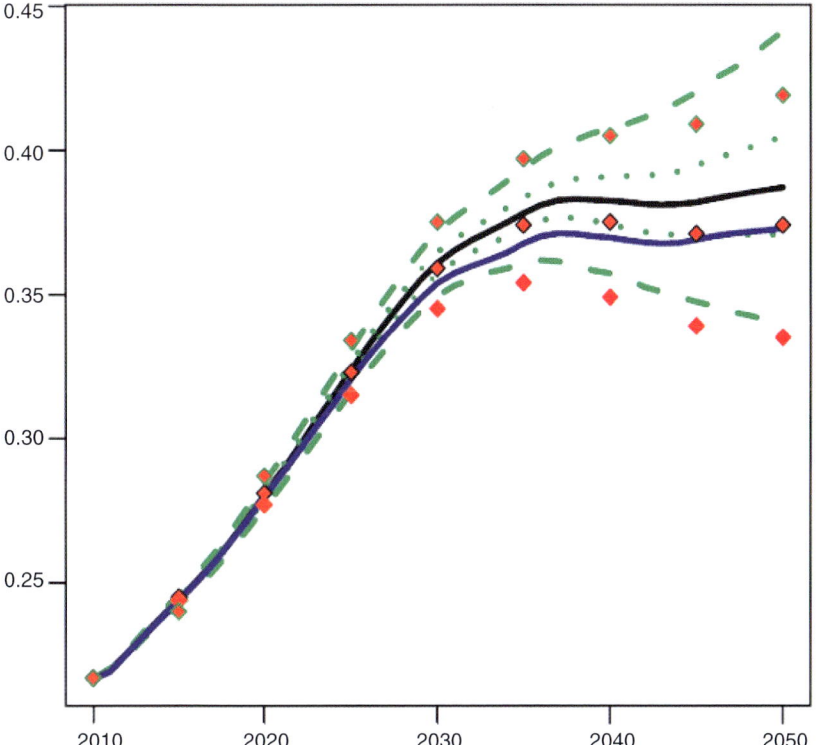

FIGURE 3-18 Old-age dependency ratio as projected by the committee, the Census Bureau, and the Social Security Trustees, 2010-2050. The central black line is the median committee forecast. There is a 50 percent probability that the ratio will lie between the green dotted lines in any year and a 95 percent probability that it will lie between the green dashed lines. The solid purple line is the 2008 Census Bureau projection. The red diamonds indicate the high, intermediate, and low variants of the 2012 Social Security Trustees projection. SOURCES: Donehower and Boe (2012), U.S. Census Bureau (2008), and Board of Trustees, Federal Old-Age and Survivors Insurance and Federal Disability Insurance Trust Funds (2012).

which 1,000 stochastic trajectories were created (see Appendix A for a description of the method used). The solid black line is the median in each year of the 1,000 random trajectories. The inner dotted green lines indicate quartiles, so there is a 50 percent chance that the future outcome will lie between them in a given year. The outer dashed green lines represent the upper and lower 2.5 percent bounds and define the 95 percent probability interval for the OADR in each year.

Figure 3-18 also plots the most recent Census Bureau projection of the OADR as a purple line. It is just at or below the lower 25 percent bound of the committee forecast, perhaps because the life expectancy forecast in the Census Bureau projection is lower than in the committee's. The Census projection does not come with a range. Figure 3-18 further shows the OADR as projected by the Social Security Trustees in its 2012 high, intermediate, and low-cost variants, all indicated by diamonds. The intermediate projection is very close to the committee's median through 2030, and then transits to the Census Bureau projection at the lower 25 percent of the committee's range. The Trustees' low-cost scenario is slightly below the lower 2.5 percent bound for the committee's forecast, while the high-cost scenario rises above the committee's upper 2.5 bound before dipping below this bound around 2040. The Trustees' projection is centered a bit lower than the committee's owing to less projected gain in longevity (life expectancy of 82.2 years in 2050, versus the committee projection of 84.5 years, as discussed earlier). The Trustees do not assign a probability to the range for the OADR, but Figure 3-18 suggests that its probability coverage is about 95 percent. This is the probability that the OADR in any given year will fall between the high-cost and low-cost brackets. This does not mean, however, that there is a 5 percent chance that the OADR would generally lie outside this range in every year between 2010 and 2050. That probability would be far lower, because a typical trajectory of the OADR would wander around within that range, with offsetting upward and downward variations.

This last point can be seen clearly in Figure 3-19, which shows a probabilistic forecast of the weighted support ratio based on the age profiles for 2007 shown earlier in Figures 3-10 and 3-11. It uses the same 1,000 stochastic trajectories and plots 20 of them for illustrative purposes. The trajectories often can be seen to fluctuate rather than to be persistently high or low. As in Figure 3-18, the solid black line is the median projection. The dashed blue lines indicate quartiles (so there is a 50 percent chance that the future outcome will lie between them in a given year), and the dashed green lines represent the upper and lower 2.5 percent bounds and define the 95 percent probability interval. The value of the ratios has been adjusted so that the ratio in 2007 is 1.0. That is, the plotted values show the ratio relative to the ratio in 2007.[9]

The expected decline in the support ratio between 2010 and 2050 is 12 percent (the same as reported earlier in this chapter), and there is a two-

---

[9] Of course, the age profiles of labor income and consumption will change over the next four decades, and any attempt to project their future levels would involve substantial uncertainty. However, the support ratio for future years is calculated using the baseline (2007) age profiles so as to isolate the effects of demographic change. Therefore the uncertainty surrounding future values of the age profiles is irrelevant. For a discussion of the construction and use of support ratios in this context, see Cutler et al. (1990).

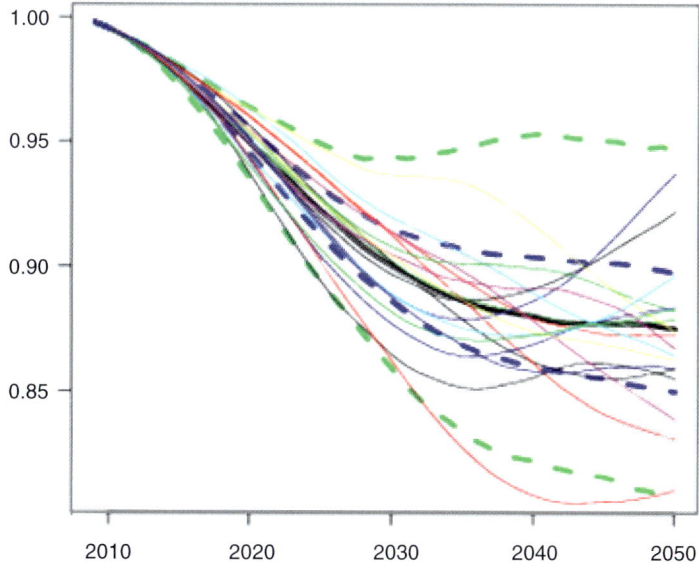

FIGURE 3-19 Projected weighted support ratio with probability bounds and 20 illustrative stochastic trajectories, 2010-2050. The central dark line is the median committee forecast. There is a 50 percent probability that the support ratio will lie between the blue dashed lines in future years and a 95 percent probability that it will lie between the green dashed lines. The figure shows 20 trajectories. The actual projection is based on 1,000 sample paths. For the method used, see Appendix A.
SOURCE: Donehower and Boe (2012).

thirds chance that the decline will be between 9 percent and 16 percent, and a 95 percent chance that it will be between 5 percent and 19 percent. We can conclude from the stochastic approach in Figures 3-18 and 3-19 that it is virtually certain that the U.S. will experience substantial population aging and that the support ratio is virtually certain to fall in the coming decades. The expected decline of 12 percent translates into an average yearly rate of decline of one-third of 1 percent (0.33 percent).

4

Health and Disability in the Working-Age and Elderly Populations

As the remarkable increases in life expectancy of the last century combined with the U.S. baby boom to cause an unprecedented demographic transformation, a fundamental question became the functional status of the future population and the pattern that would emerge in the relationship between survival and functional capacity or disability.

The functional status of the working-age and elderly populations has very significant societal and economic consequences. For while it is certainly clear that the use of health care resources increases dramatically and progressively with advancing age after age 65, these increases are seen predominantly in those with disabilities. Changes in the age-specific prevalence and severity of functional impairment might therefore be expected to have major implications for health care costs, one of the principal macroeconomic issues related to the aging of the U.S. population.

In addition, it must be emphasized that disabilities, while most common late in life, can occur at any age and that it is very important to evaluate the current trends and likely future functional status in younger cohorts as they may have an important impact on these persons' capacity to participate in the workforce and on their status as they enter late life. Thus, while the primary focus of studies of disability has been in those over 65, more recently there has been increased interest in the near elderly and younger age groups as well. Several recent studies, which will be reviewed in this chapter, shed light on these issues. Current and likely future disability rates in the so-called "young-old," those aged 65-74, are of special interest, because the future workforce may well include many individuals in this age group working part time or in flexible arrangements as a response to the later onset of social security benefits and increased workforce demands.

Recent research, reviewed in some detail in this chapter, indicates that rates of significant functional impairment for older (aged 65+) persons have been generally constant over the past decade after a two-decade period of progressive decline. Results for the "near elderly" are conflicting, probably for methodologic reasons, but there is clear evidence of the deleterious effects of increasing obesity on physical function as well as the well-documented beneficial effects of education and stopping smoking.

DISABILITY

Disability, generally defined as a limitation in the capacity to perform a given function, is traditionally considered in the framework of a process of disablement in which specific physiologic and pathophysiologic processes advance over time, resulting ultimately in a disability (Nagi, 1965; Verbrugge and Jette, 1994; Martin, Schoeni and Andreski, 2010). Various points along this spectrum may be identified. For instance the earliest stage is marked by the presence of preclinical markers, such as measures of inflammation or altered physiologic control such as high weight, blood pressure, or cholesterol. These risk factors may be followed by the presence of an identifiable disease, such as arthritis, hypertension, diabetes, heart disease, or peripheral vascular disease, which can progress.

In arthritis, for instance, the earliest clinical signs may be very subtle, though biomarkers can be identified as demonstrating risk. As the disease progresses, one advances from joint stiffness and pain to actual difficulty performing tasks and ultimately to disability.

Reasoning that the same underlying secular changes in lifestyle (smoking cessation, more exercise, public health advances, etc.) and advances in the detection and treatment of disease and physiologic risk factors such as hypercholesterolemia that led to increases in life expectancy would also naturally delay the onset of functional impairment, many expected that increases in life expectancy would be yoked to stasis or reductions in late-life disability, leading to the "compression of morbidity" concept popularized by Fries (1980). The result would be an absolute increase in active life expectancy and a progressively shorter portion of the life span spent disabled. On the other hand, some have argued that technological advances in the treatment of disease might convert some once-fatal illnesses to chronic illnesses, increasing the duration of disability as life expectancy increases.

Common Measures of Functional Capacity and Disability

Traditional measures of disability in the population have been collected in national surveys of well-defined populations for many years. The major measures include the ability or inability to perform a function as well as the difficulty of performing it and the ability to perform it without assistance. The principal metrics employed in long-term, large-scale national studies include

- *Activities of daily living (ADL).* These tasks required to take care of oneself, such as bathing, toileting, eating, and dressing, are usually measured as difficulty performing them or receiving help in performing them. These are measures of fairly severe disability and predict need for personal care services and residence in a nursing facility for long-term care.
- *Instrumental activities of daily living (IADL).* These tasks associated with the capacity to live independently, such as cooking, shopping, managing finances, and using communication devices, are measures of moderately severe disability and predict need for assistance such as homemaker and home health assistance.
- *Physical limitations in activity.* Examples are the ability to climb stairs, walk ¼ mile, stand or sit for prolonged periods, raise a 10 lb object over one's head, climb steps, stoop, bend or kneel, grasp small objects, and move large objects. These limitations may reflect underlying disease and may predict capacity to participate in certain occupations.
- *Cognitive function.* While many aspects of behavior and cognitive function change with age, including speed of processing, changes in various vocabulary subsets, decision making, and the like, most surveys evaluating functional impairment have focused on general mental status, including orientation to time and place, working memory, attention, language, calculation, and familiarity with current affairs. For most cognitive measures that decline with age, studies show the declines to be very modest until at least age 70 and, in most cases, age 75. Thus the impact on the likelihood that this age group will participate in the workforce is minimal. Recently, Skirbekk, Loichinger, and Weber (2012) proposed the use of a cognitive-function-based measure—the cognition-adjusted dependency ratio (CAGR)—as a measure of aging in populations that avoids the pitfalls of simple age-based ratios such as an old-age dependency ratio and measures based purely on physical function.

The measurement of disability is evolving. There has been growing interest in the development of additional measures of disability that account for technological change—for instance, individuals who previously were considered to have IADL disability because they could not shop or pay bills can now do these things online—and are more sensitive to the impact of the environment on functional capacity, including factors that restrict participation in activities. There has been interest as well in measuring a broader range of functional ability. Accordingly, a set of new self-reported measures has been developed and validated and will first be deployed in the emerging National Health and Aging Trends Study (Freedman et al., 2011). In addition, the Census Bureau's Survey of Income and Program Participation has recently updated its module on disability, adding new measures related to communication, ability to function independently, and a variety of measures of physical functioning.

With respect to disease states, depression is by far the most common mental disorder that influences work and home life. Over 4 percent of Americans are estimated to suffer clinically significant depression during their life, with the disorder being twice as common in women as in men and peaking in prevalence in the 25-44 year age group (Elinson et al., 2004).

Databases

With some exceptions, analyses of functional status in community-based populations have relied on one or more of the following five nationally representative longitudinal survey-based datasets:

- The Health and Retirement Study (HRS), a panel survey conducted every 2 years beginning in 1992, focuses on people aged 51 and older living in the community. Functional measures include ADL, IADL, and mobility.
- The Medicare Current Beneficiary Survey (MCBS), a panel survey of Medicare beneficiaries, includes measures of ADL and IADL.
- The National Health Interview Survey (NHIS), an annual cross-sectional household survey (one person responds with information on all household members) of the community-dwelling population, includes measures of ADL and IADL.
- The National Long Term Care Survey (NLTCS), a nationally representative panel study of the population aged 65 and older living in the community or in institutions. The survey, which began in 1982 and was repeated at regular intervals until its termination in 2004, included measures of ADL and IADL.
- The National Health and Nutrition Examination Survey (NHANES), an annual (since 1999) survey of about 5,000 adults and children, includes questions about the difficulty of performing ADL and IADL for those aged 60 and older.

Factors That Influence the Onset and Course of Disability

Disability is best seen as a function of the interaction of people's physical capacity with demands presented by their life situation and a number of lifestyle, social, and environmental factors that influence their ability to perform a task. Technology also has an important impact on disability in many ways. This goes beyond the obvious benefits of assistive devices (hearing aids, glasses, hip replacements) and includes aspects of everyday life. As noted earlier, individuals who previously were considered disabled in terms of shopping, one of the traditional IADL measures, may now shop online and are thus no longer considered to have this disability. The built environment can also be important as the absence of stairs or the presence of elevators, ramps, or electric wheelchairs can dramatically improve mobility (Freedman et al., 2006; Crimmins and Beltrán-Sánchez, 2011). Lastly but important, social activity has been shown to have a "dose-dependent" favorable impact on the development of ADL or IADL disabilities (James et al., 2011).

Biomedical Factors

Biomedical factors independent of the disease process may increase or decrease the likelihood of disability at any given level of disease severity. For instance, individuals with lung disease or peripheral vascular disease will generally have their symptoms and disability increased if they smoke. And many initially obese patients with hip and knee arthritis find improvements with weight loss. Many obese patients seem to avoid heart disease despite the presence of biomedical risk factors like high blood pressure and high cholesterol as these factors are very commonly treated with effective pharmacologic agents (Martin, Schoeni, and Andreski, 2010).

The development of disability is a potentially reversible process. Clearly certain technologies such as hip or knee replacements or cataract removal promise dramatic reductions in disability, as do the less dramatic treatment of many diseases and many of the technologic, lifestyle, or environmental changes mentioned above. Such treatments can also increase the prevalence of disability in the population. For instance, changes in lifestyle (smoking, exercise) and improved treatment of risk factors (high blood pressure, high cholesterol) have decreased the incidence of stroke and, more recently, heart attack and some forms of cancer, reducing mortality and increasing survivorship and the prevalence of these disorders (Crimmins and Beltrán-Sánchez, 2011).

While it has been developing over several decades, the "obesity epidemic" (especially among certain racial and socioeconomic groups) has recently begun to attract widespread attention. Increases in weight beyond the "normal" range, whether of moderate degree (overweight) or more marked (obese), have long been associated with increases in a number of important biomedical risk factors such as blood lipids, blood pressure, and blood sugar and have been shown to increase the risk for diabetes and a number of forms of cancer and cardiovascular disease. Over the last 30 years of the twentieth century, the prevalence of overweight tripled among children and adolescents while the prevalence of obesity in adults doubled to reach 33 percent (Ogden et al., 2007). Evidence is accumulating that this steady decades-long increase may have abated, as obesity and overweight rates seem to have flattened over the past decade (Ogden et al., 2006 and 2007; Martin, Schoeni, and Andreski, 2010).

Despite the widespread concern about obesity, some observers note that the adverse impact may be exaggerated in the media. Like many risk factors, the effect of increasing weight seems dose-related, with the greatest effects at extreme levels and only modest effects at low levels, despite the fact that such individuals may be labeled overweight or even obese (Wee et al., 2011). In addition, many of the metabolic risk factors associated with obesity, such as hypercholesterolemia, are now being effectively managed with medications, and the cardiovascular risk profile of today's overweight and obese individuals may be improving. As Martin, Schoeni, and Andreski (2010) say, "Thus, for a variety of reasons, what it means to be obese may be changing, possibly for the better, over time." A number of biomedical factors, including reductions in smoking, a plateau in the prevalence of obesity, and mitigation of its adverse effects through management, all point to positive changes in biomedically mediated disability in the future.

EDUCATION AND INCOME

Socioeconomic status (SES) has long been recognized as a major predictor of mortality, health status, and disability. The SES effect appears early in life and persists in a graded fashion so that advantage accrues as one "climbs the SES ladder" (Kawachi, Adler, and Dow, 2010). In most analyses education has been used as a proxy for socioeconomic status, which includes income and social status.

Analyses of the independent effects of education are complicated by the obvious selection effects (education is not randomly distributed) and by the clear confound with income, and studies that have tried to disentangle the two have generally shown that they have independent effects. Thorough analyses by Cutler and Lleras-Muney (2006 and 2010) conclude that the health-education gradient is found both for health behaviors and for health status and suggest that cognitive ability and decision-making patterns explain a large portion of the gradient. The effect of education on delaying the onset of disability is robust, dose-dependent, and present across the lifespan (Taylor, 2010) (Figure 4-1). In addition to leading to higher income and professional status, thus providing greater access to health care, health insurance, and technological and personnel assistance, there are a number of other pathways by which education might influence the onset or course of disability, including enhancement of psychosocial resources, lifestyle differences (smoking, exercise), presence of fewer stressors such as marital or legal problems, and occupational factors—for example, more-educated individuals are less likely to be exposed to the risks of injury common in agricultural, commercial fishing, and construction work.

Since the beginning of the twentieth century there has been a very significant increase in educational attainment in the United States in successive cohorts of elderly (Figure 4-2). This secular change in education has been an important driver of changes in disability.

Poverty poses special risks as it is associated with significant increases in many biological risk factors for ill health and disability, especially during midlife. Poverty is related to not only the onset but also the course of disability, leading to the widely accepted view that the poor may age as much as a decade sooner than those who are well off (Crimmins, Kim, and Seeman, 2009; Taylor, 2010) (Figure 4-3). Regardless of the specific pathways operational in a given individual or group, it is abundantly clear that well-educated, high-income individuals are at greater advantage regarding survival and functional capacity while relatively uneducated, poor individuals are at greater relative risk.

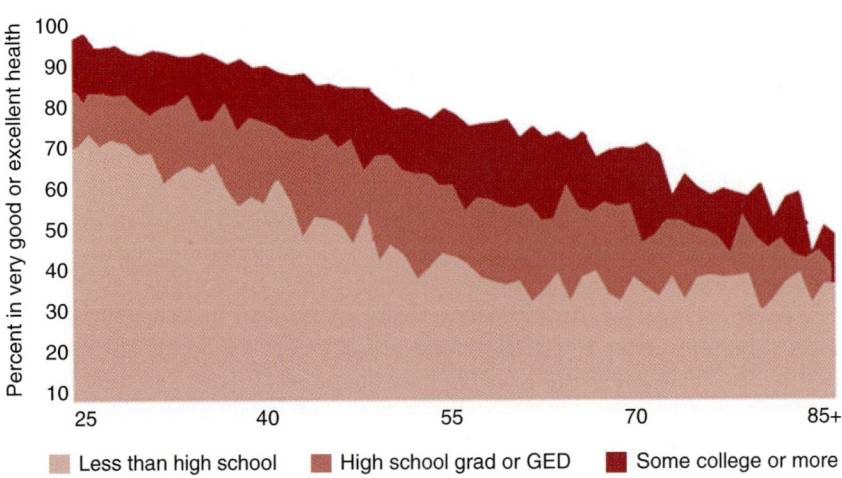

FIGURE 4-1 Age, education, and functional decline, 2002-2004. SOURCE: MacArthur Foundation Research Network on an Aging Society (2009), based on data from the National Health Interview Survey.

HEALTH AND DISABILITY

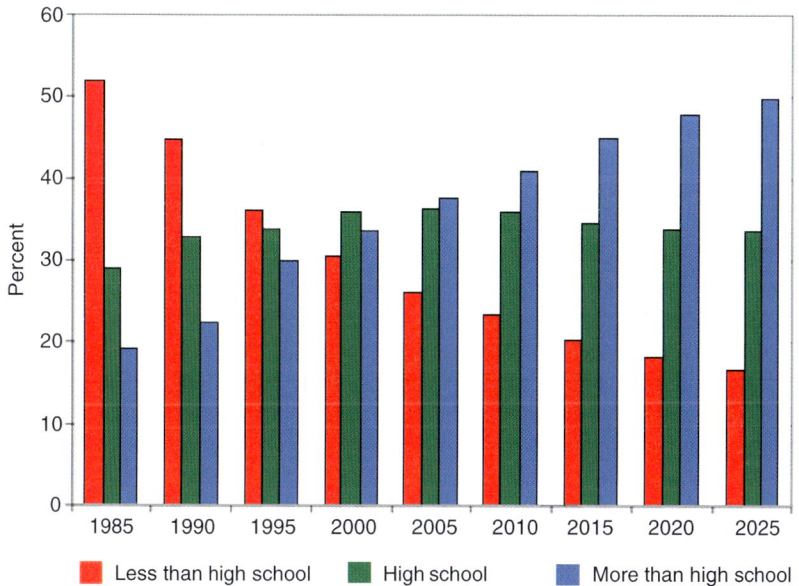

FIGURE 4-2 Educational attainment at ages 65+, 1985 to 2025. SOURCE: Martin, Schoeni, and Andreski (2010).

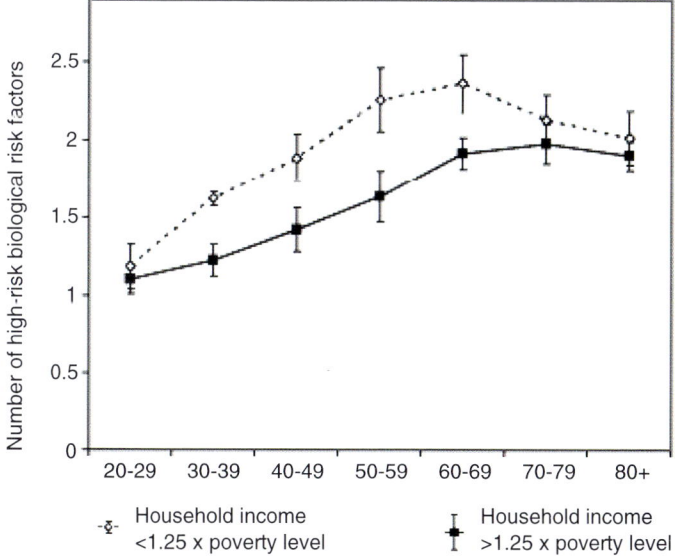

FIGURE 4-3 Mean number of high-risk biological risk factors, by poverty status and age, 1999-2004. SOURCE: Crimmins, Kim, and Seeman (2009). Reprinted by permission.

TRENDS IN DISABILITY

Working Age Population

As mentioned previously, the future workforce may include more individuals between the ages of 65 and 75 years. For this reason, and to better understand likely future disability trends in older persons, there has been a recent increase in interest in studying functional capacity in nonelderly adults, especially those over 40 years of age. In addition, an important advance has been the extension of measures of function beyond the traditional ADL/IADL to measures of less severe disability, such as mobility, which may not influence use of health care resources but may have an important impact on the capacity of persons to work in certain occupations.

With respect to moderate or severe limitations of function in nonelderly individuals, several studies have indicated that rates of fair/poor self-rated health or of severe disability (ADL/IADL) for the near elderly have been gradually increasing over the past decade or two at a rate of about 1-2 percent per decade (Box 4-1). About 3-5 percent of near elderly report that they require help with either ADL or IADL (Figure 4-4), with as many as 14-16 percent reporting that they can perform these tasks alone but with difficulty (Freedman et al., 2011; Martin et al., 2009; Bhattacharya, Choudhry, and Lakdawalla, 2008).

Crimmins and Beltrán-Sánchez, using the National Health Interview Survey database and defining limitations as difficulty in any of four fairly robust functional measures (walking a quarter mile, climbing a flight of steps, standing or sitting for 2 hours, and bending or kneeling), found an increase in the prevalence of limitations in physical functioning that might be seen as reflecting less severe disability than ADL or IADL in middle age in all age groups between 1998 and 2006. For example, the limitation rate rose from 6.3 to 7.9 percent for men aged 50-59, and from 10.7 to 15.6 percent for men aged 60-69. Rates for women were higher than for men at all ages.

In contradiction to these findings, Martin, Schoeni, and Andreski (2010), using data from the NHIS for 1997-2008, found no changes over time in the proportion of people aged 40-64 who display difficulty in physical function. It should be noted that this study employed a much less strict measure of functional impairment (difficulty with any of nine measures, including walking a quarter mile, climbing 10 steps, standing 2 hours, sitting 2 hours, stooping, bending, or kneeling, reaching over one's head, grasping small objects, and carrying 10 pounds or moving large objects) than did Crimmins and Beltrán-Sánchez. In unpacking the effects of various factors over time, Martin, Schoeni, and Andreski found that the stability in

> **BOX 4-1**
> **The Economics of Disability**
>
> Key questions are why so many Americans are currently classified as disabled and why the incidence of disability has risen so quickly in the past three decades. In 1970, for instance, the proportion of beneficiaries of the government-run Disability Insurance (DI) program was below 3 percent; today it has risen to over 5 percent, and by 2030 is projected to be almost 7 percent (Social Security Administration, 2011). A partial explanation for the substantial run-up in the incidence of disability is the fact that Congress made it easier for those with mental illness and back pain to receive benefits.[a] Moreover, since people with these problems tend to live relatively long, the size of the disabled population has risen. Another explanation is that both the financial and in-kind benefits provided by the DI program have increased over time, making it more attractive for workers to apply than in the past. In addition, the rise in women's labor market attachment has also raised the number of DI-insured workers, making it possible for more workers to claim benefits. Virtually none of the rise in DI receipt can be attributable to population aging or declining health (Autor and Duggan, 2006).
>
> Future disability policy will surely have a powerful effect on labor force attachment patterns of Americans, because so many people are receiving benefits and because the financial flows associated with the DI program are so substantial. Policy makers coping with shortfalls in the nation's safety net programs will need to carefully consider how generous the programs can be while at the same time encouraging employment among those who can work. Moreover, means of disability prevention also deserve more attention (Burkhauser and Daly, 2011).
>
> ---
>
> [a]For in-depth studies of the American disability system and proposals for change, see Autor and Duggan, 2006; Haveman and Wolfe, 2000; and Burkhauser and Daly, 2011.

reported disability resulted from a balance between the adverse effects of increasing obesity and the benefits of declining smoking rates.

The Elderly

One of the strongest and most durable findings in disability research was the significant progressive reduction in functional impairment that occurred in older Americans from the 1980s into the early 2000s (Figure 4-5). Reductions in disability were prominent with respect to IADL but also were found, to a lesser extent, in ADL, indicating that both moderate and severe disability rates were falling (Schoeni, Freedman, and Martin, 2008; Freedman et al., 2004, Seeman et al., 2010). As discussed previously, medical advances and progressive increases in social factors, including education, likely mediated many of these improvements. As summarized by Freed-

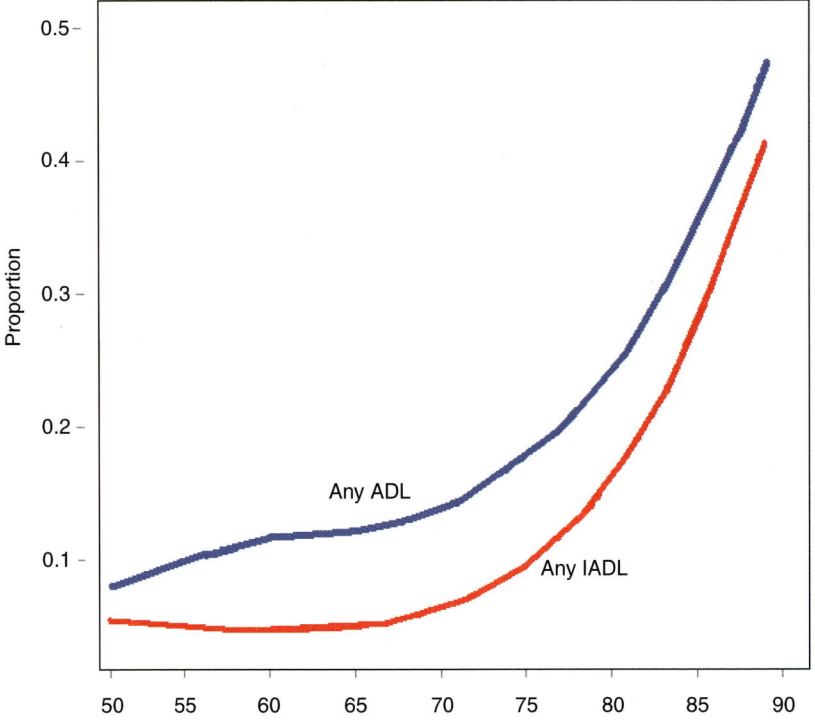

FIGURE 4-4 Proportion of people aged 50-89 requiring help with one or more ADL or IADL, 2004. SOURCE: Data from Health and Retirement Study.

man (2011), these trends resulted in increases in active life expectancy and "compression of morbidity" during the 1980s and 1990s.

During the last decade, however, the picture has become quite murky, with disparate results and methodologic questions leading to uncertainty about whether these improvements were continuing. Recently several leading scholars in the area joined together in a robust analysis of all five of the large-scale databases noted earlier to evaluate trends in the functioning of older persons during the period 2000 to 2008. In general, the most consistent finding from this analysis was the lack of significant change in ADL or IADL for the 65- to 85-year-old population. For those over 85 the previous reductions in ADL seem to have continued, especially if one includes the nursing home population. This likely reflects continued increases in educational attainment in successive over-85-year-old cohorts during this time (Freedman et al., in press). The current prevailing view is that the period

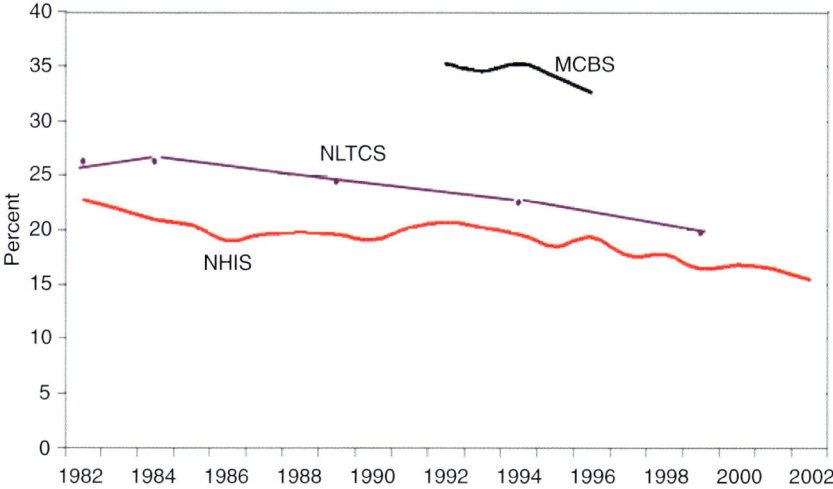

FIGURE 4-5 Trend in disability rate for ages 65+ in three national surveys.
SOURCE: Data as reported in the MCBS, the NLTCS, and the NHIS.

of declining ADL/IADL disability in older persons ended in the beginning of the last decade.

When it comes to less severe forms of disability, such as limitations in movement and the like, a different picture may be emerging. Using data from NHANES and NHIS, Martin, Schoeni, and Andreski (2010) found that two-thirds of the elderly had a limitation in at least one of the nine physical functions listed earlier. From 1997 to 2008 this prevalence was stable for males and increased gradually (1 percent per year) for females. The authors found, as did others who work in this area, that the effect of education was important and that the increase in educational attainment for the elderly during this time mitigated what would otherwise have been an increase in the prevalence of these limitations.

LOOKING FORWARD

The leveling off of disability decline in the older population, combined with apparent increases in disability among the working age population, complicates the forecasting of disability and related health care costs. In addition, other sources of uncertainty deserve mention. On the one hand, things could get worse than expected. Certain secular changes, such as the dramatic increase in overweight and obesity among the nonelderly and the tendency for underprivileged populations to drop out of school, suggest that future generations may fare less well than their predecessors in this regard. Difficult-to-treat infectious diseases continue to emerge and could have a significant impact, especially later in life. What is more, the increasing political and economic pressures on entitlement programs that provide financial security and health care for older persons and the poor may have significant effects on their access to health care.

On the other hand, things could get much better. Continued advances in biomedicine, especially a cure for cancer or Alzheimer's disease, could have remarkable effects, as would basic advances that slow the process of aging, which remains the major risk factor for disability. Of course, the committee is not interested in disability for its own sake but rather for its effect on the need for personal care services and its impact on the capacity of individuals to work. This latter consideration includes both those in the traditional "working age" category as well as those over 64 who may wish or need to work. In the next chapter the committee presents forecasts it commissioned of the size of the future workforce, including individuals up to age 74, based on several possible trajectories of disability change.

5

Labor Force Participation and Retirement

Chapter 3 discusses the aging of the U.S. population and the accompanying increase in average life expectancy. The macroeconomic implications of these demographic trends will depend in large part on the future growth of the labor force and on how long people stay in the labor force. Working longer can provide more resources to pay for the higher Social Security and health care costs associated with population aging. It will also allow a smaller proportion of total resources to be used for support of the older population and more to be allocated to the young, to education in particular. How long people work will depend on health and disability trends, the incentive effects of public and private pension programs, the demand for older workers, and the flexibility of work at older ages.

The first part of this chapter describes trends in the labor force since 1950 and projections for future years and discusses the changing job mix and changing human capital needs. The chapter then explores trends in employment by health status and the capacity to work at older ages and examines public and private policies that induce early retirement. The discussion concludes with a look at ways that longer working lives can be facilitated and summarizes the macroimplications of longer working lives.

TRENDS IN LABOR FORCE SIZE, PARTICIPATION, AND PROJECTIONS

Labor Force Size and Composition

Changes in labor force size and composition in the United States over the past 60 years may be attributed to three main trends. The first, as described in Chapter 3, was the overall growth of the population after the Second World War. Beginning in the early 1960s, the surge in labor force size was propelled by the large number of postwar babies who began to enter the labor force. A second contributor to labor force growth was the increase in the number and proportion of women, especially married women, undertaking employment. The third factor was an increase in the number foreign-born workers, which accelerated in the 1970s.

Between 1950 and 2010, the labor force[1] grew more rapidly than did the population as a whole. Whereas the total U.S. population increased 102 percent over the 60-year period, the corresponding increase in civilian labor force size was 148 percent. The highest rates of labor force growth were seen in the 1970s, when large numbers of the baby boom generation entered the prime working ages (Figure 5-1). By the 1980s, the majority of the baby boomers were of working age. While the absolute size of the labor force has continued to rise since the 1970s, the decadal growth rates have declined.

Non-Hispanic whites constitute the bulk of the total labor force (70 percent in 2005), but the racial and ethnic composition of workers has been changing. The proportion of the labor force that is foreign-born increased from 6 percent in 1960 to 13 percent in 2000 and to 16 percent in 2009 (Lee and Mather, 2008; Bureau of Labor Statistics, 2011b).

Labor Force Participation

The long-term growth of the labor force has been the product of several subtrends, not all of which have moved in the same direction. The total labor force participation rate (people aged 16 and over in the labor force as a percent of the civilian noninstitutional population aged 16 and over) fluctuated between 58 and 60 percent in the 1950s and the first half of the 1960s. Beginning in the mid-1960s, the labor force participation rate (LFPR) began a long-term increase that reached a high point—67 percent—in the latter 1990s. The LFPR declined slightly, to 66 percent in the mid-2000s and less than 65 percent in 2010.

Figure 5-2 indicates the labor force participation experience of four broad age/sex groupings. Men have always constituted the majority of the U.S. labor force, but as the total labor force has grown over the past 60 years, the participation rate of prime age (25-54) men has declined some-

---

[1] The Bureau of Labor Statistics defines "labor force" to include all persons aged 16 or older in the civilian, noninstitutionalized population who, during a given reference week, (1) worked as paid employees or in their own business, (2) worked 15 hours or more without pay in a family enterprise, (3) were temporarily absent from a regular job, or (4) had no employment but were available for work, except for temporary illness, and had made specific efforts to find employment sometime during the 4-week period ending with the reference week.

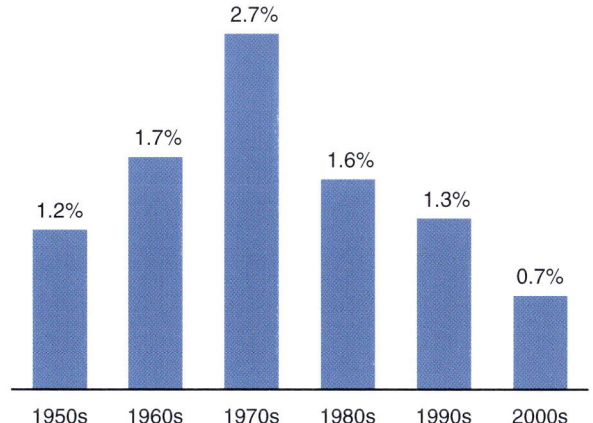

FIGURE 5-1 Average annual labor force growth, by decade, 1950s to 2000s. SOURCE: Bureau of Labor Statistics.

what. More striking is the decline in the participation rate from 1950 to 1995 among men aged 55 and over, from nearly 70 percent to less than 40 percent. This drop reflects the declines in average age at retirement (discussed below) that occurred since the 1950s, a pattern also seen throughout most of the industrialized world. Since the mid-1990s, however, the partici-

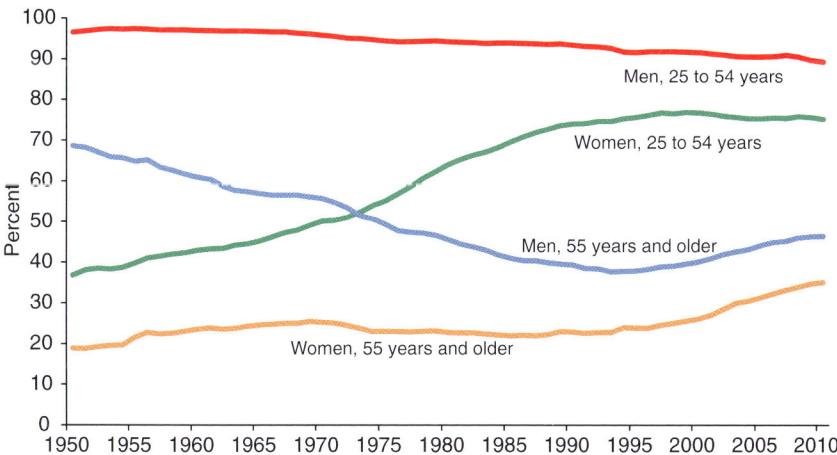

FIGURE 5-2 Labor force participation rates for four broad age-sex groups, 1950-2011. SOURCE: Bureau of Labor Statistics.

pation rate among older men has reversed course and now approaches 50 percent, even as the overall LFPR was flat or declining.

Trends among women were distinctly different from those for men, at least between 1950 and 2000. The combination of economic growth and changing social norms produced a surge in female labor force participation rates during the second half of the twentieth century; the participation rate for women aged 25-54 doubled between 1950 and 2000, before declining slightly in the first decade of the 2000s. The participation rate for older women, unlike that for older men, rose from 1950 to 1970 and was essentially stable during the following two decades. After 1995, there was an upward trend for older women similar to that for older men.

Figure 5-3 takes a closer look at trends at older ages from 1976 to 2011. For men, it can be seen that the aggregate gains at ages 55 and over since the mid-1990s were driven mainly by increased participation at ages 60-64 and 65-69, with little change at ages 55-59. Increases in participation among women were seen in all older age groups. Note that LFPRs at ages 70 and over are not insignificant: more than 15 percent for men and 8 percent for women in 2011. And in spite of the economic downturn in 2008-2009, the total LFPR of people aged 55 and over continued to increase. This upturn seems likely to continue, at least in the near future, as people (1) work additional years to recoup assets that were lost owing to declining stock values and (2) seek to maintain access to employment-based health coverage (Copeland, 2011).

While participation rates vary by race and ethnic group, the differences are not as large as the variance seen across age and sex categories (Toossi, 2006). Since at least the mid-1970s, participation rates for Hispanic men have been somewhat higher than for white men and black men. Data from the mid-1970s through 2006 showed that the LFPR for Hispanic men averaged 81 percent, compared with 77 percent for whites and 70 percent for blacks (DiCecio et al., 2008). The relatively high level for Hispanic men reflects the fact that Hispanic men are younger, on average, than the overall population—that is, they are more likely to be in age groups that have the highest activity rates. The picture for women was quite different; the average LFPR for Hispanic women was 52 percent, lower than that for white women (55 percent) and black women (57 percent).

Projections of the Labor Force

The interplay between future demographic and labor force characteristics is a key factor in any macroeconomic assessment of aging. The committee considers changes in the size of the labor force and participation rates and likely changes in the composition of the labor force through 2050. The committee developed its own labor force projections as an adjunct to the

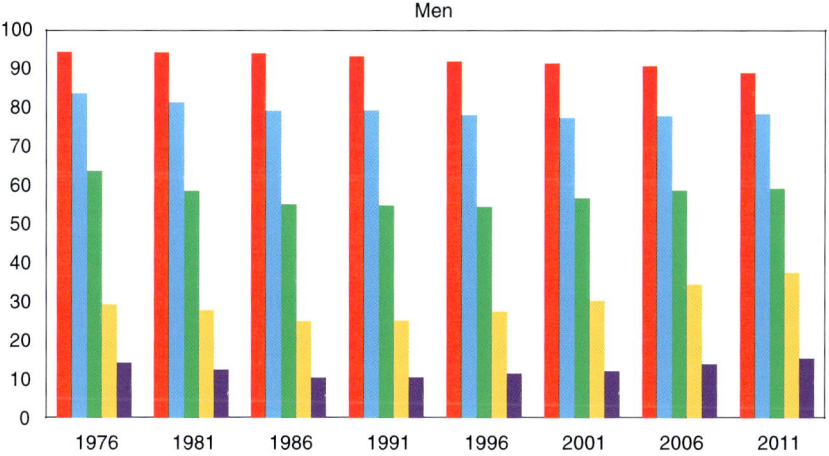

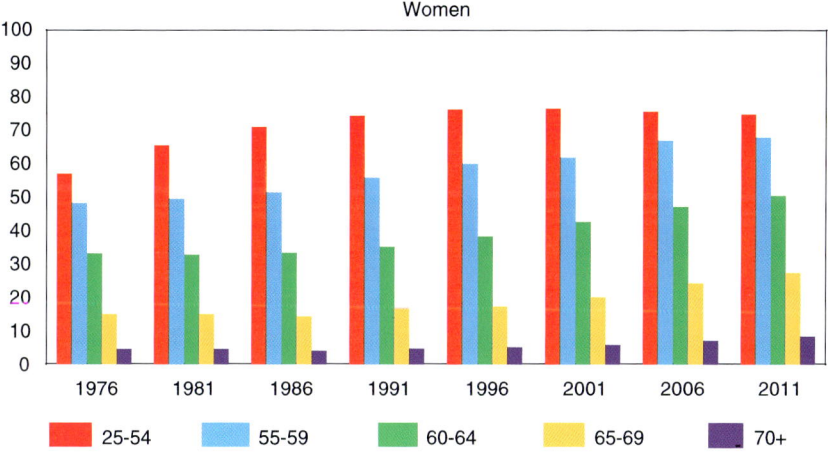

FIGURE 5-3 Labor force participation rates for prime-age and older workers, 1976-2011. SOURCE: Bureau of Labor Statistics.

population projections presented in Chapter 3 (see Appendix A for details). Data from the Bureau of Labor Statistics (BLS) and the Census Bureau's Current Population Survey were used to add a race/ethnic group component to the population projections. The resulting labor force projections suggest that the growth rate of the labor force will be essentially flat from 2010 to 2015 and will then resume the downward trend seen in Figure 5-1. The overall annual labor force growth rate is projected to decline from 0.69 to 0.50 between 2015 and 2027, then increase to 0.63 by 2040 before declining slightly to 0.60 by 2050. This overall trend reflects the interplay of several factors:

- The labor force will continue to age as the overall U.S. population ages. The median age of workers rose from less than 35 years in 1980 to more than 40 in 2010; the median age is projected to approach 41 by 2015 and increase gradually to 42 during the following 25 years. Other things being equal, the entrance of large baby boom cohorts into age groups that traditionally have lower LFPRs should exert a downward force on the overall LFPR.
- The share of young (16-24) workers in the total labor force is likely to decline throughout the entire 2010-2050 period, from 14 percent to 11 percent.
- The share of prime-age (25-54) workers in the total labor force is projected to decline, from 66 percent in 2010 to 62 percent in 2027, then rise slightly for 6 years before declining to 61 percent in 2050.
- The declining share of workers aged 16-54 will be offset by an increasing percentage of all workers who are aged 55 and above. The latter share was 12 percent in 1990, is projected to double to 24 percent around 2020, and should rise to more than 27 percent by 2050.

As the age distribution of the labor force changes, the racial and ethnic composition of the labor force is likely to become increasingly diverse. The committee projects an average annual growth rate of 2.2 percent and 1.7 percent for the Hispanic and Asian components of the labor force, respectively, from 2010 to 2050. In contrast, the average annual growth of the black component is expected to be 0.6 percent, while the white component is expected to decline by 0.1 percent annually over the 40-year period. The white non-Hispanic share of the total labor force is expected to decline from two-thirds in 2010 to about half by 2050 (67 to 51 percent). In addition to the differential growth rates by race and ethnicity, the white non-Hispanic share also will decline because of (1) lower fertility of white non-Hispanics relative to other population groups, which means proportionally fewer white non-Hispanic workers in the future, and (2) the eventual retirement of the largely white, non-Hispanic baby boom (Toossi, 2006).

Female Labor Force Participation and Fertility

Long-term projections of the size and composition of the nation's labor force depend on several key variables, including female labor force participation (FLFP). As mentioned earlier, women's participation in the labor force increased steadily during much of the latter half of the twentieth century. Whereas 33 percent of women aged 16 years or older reported working in 1948, this figure had reached 60 percent (an all-time high) by the turn of the century. Over the last 25 years, much of the increase in FLFP has occurred among mothers with newborn children (Martinez and Iza, 2004). Women represented 47 percent of the total U.S. labor force in 2009 and are expected to account for more than half of the increase in total labor force growth through 2018 (Department of Labor, 2010).

While historical data highlight the dramatic changes in FLFP during the twentieth century, figures over the past 15 years indicate a plateau. By 2007, FLFP had decreased to its 1996 level of 59 percent (Vere, 2007). It is unclear whether this represents a long-term trend or a temporary stagnation in FLFP. Predicting FLFP—and, by extension, the characteristics of the labor force as a whole—relies on understanding several factors that could influence FLFP in the coming years.

Returns to female laborers have increased in absolute and relative terms since the early twentieth century and have been a driving factor behind women's entry into the labor market (Galor and Weil, 1996). Today, women aged 25-34 are more likely than men to finish high school, obtain a college degree, and obtain a graduate degree. Thus, women are increasingly well qualified to enter the workforce at all skill levels. Though gender disparities in pay persist, they continue to narrow. In 2009, women earned approximately 80 percent of men's weekly earnings, compared with 62 percent in 1979 (White House Council on Women and Girls, 2011). Further change in compensation may spur continued growth in FLFP.

The relationship between fertility (childbearing) and FLFP has been the subject of considerable investigation in recent decades. A negative relationship between FLFP and childbearing has been well documented in many countries. However, in spite of less generous family policies, the United States has relatively high levels of fertility and female labor market participation compared with other developed nations. Moreover, research suggests that the magnitude and significance of the trade off between work and children has lessened in the United States since the 1980s (Furtado and Hock, 2008; Engelhardt and Prskawetz, 2004).

Several factors besides enhanced wage incentives could be responsible for the changing nature of the relationship between FLFP and fertility in the United States. Increased divorce rates, labor-saving household technologies, and declines in real wages for some groups of male workers have been identified as possible explanations for increased FLFP (Juhn and Potter, 2006). The influx of low-skilled immigrant workers is thought to have increased the affordability of child care for relatively higher-skilled workers (Furtado and Hock, 2010; Martinez and Iza, 2004). It also has been noted that increased social, political, and legal support for working mothers has lessened the conflict between paid work and family responsibilities. For instance, the enactment of the 1993 Family and Medical Leave Act and the introduction of child care subsidies helped to increase both job security and labor force participation for working mothers (Apps and Rees, 2004; Brewster and Rindfuss, 2000). Further, federal programs such as Temporary Assistance for Needy Families (TANF) and the Earned Income Tax Credit (EITC), which provide an incentive for work or require work in exchange for state and federal assistance, have encouraged low-skilled workers to enter the labor force.

Part-Time Work

Societal responses to an unfavorable worker/retiree support ratio could involve incentives for older workers to remain in the labor force longer, as discussed at some length later in this chapter. One such incentive is the option of part-time work, which may facilitate gradual or phased retirement. Phased retirement in the United States appears to be gaining popularity among both employers and employees, notably in areas that have a current or projected shortage of workers (e.g., public school teachers and administrators) (Watson Wyatt Worldwide, 2004; Chen and Scott, 2006; Purcell, 2009b). Legislative changes have sought to ease restrictions on older employees' receipt of pension benefits, and a congressional research report indicated that 41 percent of men and 35 percent of women aged 55-64 who reported receiving pension income in 2005 were employed in 2007 (Purcell, 2007).

Data suggest that many older workers work part-time as a transition to retirement. Part-time employment is more common among older than younger workers, and older women are more likely than older men to work part-time. In 2002, more than half of working women aged 65 who were surveyed in the Health and Retirement Study (a panel survey that began in 1992 and surveyed respondents every 2 years thereafter) were employed in part-time positions, compared with about 30 percent of men. And among older workers, the proportion working part-time increases with age; for both genders, part-time employment formed the lion's share of total employment for people aged 70 and over (National Institute on Aging, 2007). Figure 5-4 indicates that in spite of the apparent prevalence of part-time work, the proportion of older workers employed part-time has declined since the mid-1990s, with a slight uptick between 2008 and 2009.

Retirement Trends

One important issue for policy makers and pension funds is the relationship between the statutory retirement age (also called the full retirement

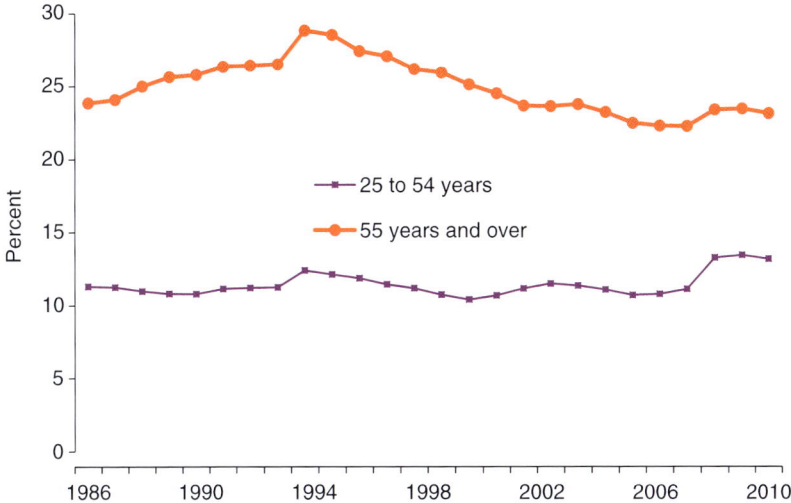

FIGURE 5-4 Share of employed individuals engaged in part-time work for two broad age groups, 1986-2011. The jump in share around 1994 is a function of a redesign of the Current Population Survey. SOURCE: Bureau of Labor Statistics.

age or normal retirement age), the age at which one can leave the labor force and receive full benefits, and the actual retirement age, the average age at which people leave the labor force and/or begin to receive some retirement benefits. The average age is heavily influenced by early retirement incentives inherent in plan provisions, as discussed later in the chapter.

There are numerous ways of defining "retirement," and different data sources yield different estimates of when people retire and how much of life is spent in retirement. For example, Gendell (2008) calculated average retirement ages of 62.6 years for men and 62.5 years for women in the early to mid-2000s using Social Security data and somewhat lower ages (61.6 and 60.5 years, respectively) using labor force data from the Current Population Survey, a joint effort between the Bureau of Labor Statistics and the Census Bureau. The Organization for Economic Co-operation and Development (OECD), using a methodology based on net withdrawals from the labor market, posited higher average retirement ages of 64.1 years for men and 63.2 years for women, circa 2003. Regardless of methodology, however, it seems clear that a greater proportion of older Americans are currently working than was the case two decades ago, as is shown in Figure 5-3. The most recent OECD calculation, for 2009, suggests an average retirement age of 65.3 for men and 64.8 for women (Organisation for Economic Co-operation and Development, 2010).[2] While the trends in average retirement age have changed in recent decades, the age at which individuals initially receive Social Security retirement benefits has remained fairly constant since 1975, averaging around 63.7 years. There is little difference in the age at which men and women initially receive Social Security retirement benefits (Social Security Administration, 2010a).

TRENDS IN JOBS AND CHANGING HUMAN CAPITAL NEEDS

It has been argued that technology may change the nature of work faster than the skills of the workforce change. In modern economies, problems abound when a nation's educational system grows out of touch with job market trends (Levy, 2010). This section takes a brief look at trends in job mix that have evolved during the past century, as well as short-term forecasts of changing occupational structure. The committee then considers the likely impact of technological change on U.S. job requirements over a longer time horizon.

Changes in the Job Mix

The distribution of U.S. workers by occupation underwent a transformation in the twentieth century, largely in response to industrialization and urbanization. Farmers and farm laborers constituted a third of the entire labor force in 1910, but their proportion had shrunk to 2 percent by 2000. Less precipitous but still large declines were seen among private household service workers, nonfarm laborers, and operatives—for example, workers who ran machines in rapidly expanding industries such as steel, paper, and chemicals. At the other end of the spectrum, the proportion of professional and technical workers jumped about 400 percent, and large proportional gains were seen for clerical workers, nonhousehold service workers, and the occupational category that includes managers, officials, and proprietors (Wyatt and Hecker, 2006).

As noted earlier, the BLS makes short-term projections of various labor force characteristics, one of which is growth among 750 detailed occupations. These occupations can be aggregated into 10 major groupings and

---

[2]The OECD calculates the average effective age of retirement as a weighted average of net withdrawals from the labor market at different ages over a 5-year period for workers initially aged 40 and over. In order to abstract from compositional effects in the age structure of the population, labor force withdrawals are estimated based on changes in labor force participation rates rather than labor force levels. These changes are calculated for each (synthetic) cohort divided into 5-year age groups. For more detail, see http://www.oecd.org/employment/employmentpoliciesanddata/39371923.pdf.

examined for variations in employment growth. The latest set of occupational projections, covering the period 2008-2018, foresees the most rapid growth (17 percent) among professional and related occupations, while production occupations will face a decline of 3.5 percent. The professional and related group is projected to account for the largest number of new jobs, in excess of 5.2 million, whereas a loss of about 350,000 positions is forecast in production occupations (Lacey and Wright, 2009). Although the general U.S. economic situation during 2009-2011 might affect any absolute numerical forecasts of job growth, it seems likely that the projected changes in job mix are realistic.

Technology and Changing Job Requirements

More detailed data from the 2008-2018 BLS projections illustrate the dual impact that technology and population aging are likely to have. The occupational category with the largest projected growth is "network systems and data communications analysts." The second and third categories are "home health aides" and "personal and home care aides," which reflect in large part the needs of an aging population. Computer software engineers and medical assistants round out the five highest projected growth areas. Data collected since these projections illustrate the importance of changes in the health sector: Private sector job changes in 13 major categories in 2009-2010 show a net job loss in each category except one: education and health services (U.S. Census Bureau, 2012).

There is little disagreement that the pace of technological change seen in recent decades will continue or accelerate. Technological advances will increase demand for a highly skilled workforce who can respond and adapt to new technologies and new product demand and grow productivity (Karoly and Panis, 2004). Numerous studies have attempted to gauge the fit between shifting employment and occupation patterns and the educational skills of U.S. workers. Separate analyses of job and education requirements in the 2010 decade, done independently from the BLS analysis, suggest that the United States will need 20-22 million new college degree holders but will fall short of that mark by at least 1.5-3.0 million degrees (Carnevale, Smith, and Strohl, 2010; Manyika et al., 2011).

During the 1990s and 2000s, the fraction of the workforce engaged in very low and very high skill occupations increased, while the fraction engaged in moderately skilled occupations contracted. Information technology (IT) is suited to highly educated workers engaged in abstract tasks and much less so to less-educated workers engaged in routine tasks. IT development has less impact on low-skilled workers engaged in manual labor (Autor, 2008; Autor and Dorn, 2011). A McKinsey Global Institute (2009) analysis suggests that 71 percent of U.S. workers are in jobs for which there is either low demand from employers or an oversupply of workers, or both. Income and employment for the top-earning fifth of the U.S. labor force grew rapidly from the mid-1990s to the mid-2000s, mainly because global changes in technology generated new market opportunities and demand for advanced skills.

TRENDS IN EMPLOYMENT BY HEALTH

The combination of increasing life expectancy and large numbers of people moving into traditional retirement ages—and until the mid 1990s the decline in the LFPRs of men in particular (Figure 5-3, top panel)—has put fiscal strains on income support programs and medical care for older people not only in the United States but also in many other countries. To ease these strains, policy discussions here and elsewhere have more and more focused on an increase in Social Security retirement ages and incentives for older individuals to remain in the labor force. An important backdrop for these discussions is that older people in general are able to work later in life than earlier generations. This section considers several metrics that bear on the capacity to work at older ages. Here the committee emphasizes measures of health and capacity to work at or near typical retirement ages. Chapter 4 gives more attention to health and disability at older ages.

Mortality and Other Measures

Figure 5-5 shows two trends. The first is the relationship between age and employment for men in 1977 and 2007 (Milligan and Wise, 2011). The employment rate by age did not change much between the two years, at least through age 64. Specifically, as highlighted by the box in Figure 5-5, the employment rate at ages 62 and 63 changed very little between 1977 and 2007. But the male mortality rate at these ages declined substantially between 1977 and 2007. For example, the mortality rate for men aged 63 was 2.6 percent in 1977 but had fallen to 1.5 percent by 2007.

Figure 5-6 presents a different view of the data. This figure shows the employment rate by mortality rate in 1977 and 2007, together with ages corresponding to selected mortality rates. For example, consider the mortality rate of 1.5 percent on the x axis. In 1977, this was the mortality rate for men at age 57, and 80 percent of men were working at that age. In 2007, 1.5 percent was the mortality rate for men at age 63, and only 50 percent of men were working at that age. In other words, the probability of being employed when the mortality rate was 1.5 percent was 0.8 in 1977 and 0.5 in 2007.[3] On average, men aged 63 worked 0.3 fewer years in 2007 than

---

[3]Looking at the data another way, consider the 50 percent employment level for men. In 1977, the mortality rate when 50 percent of men were employed was 2.7 percent; 30 years

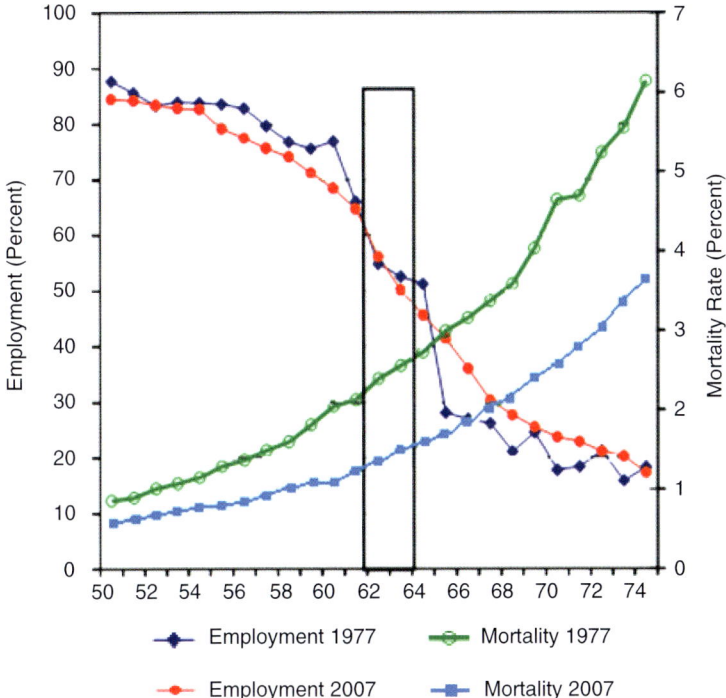

FIGURE 5-5 Male employment and mortality by age, 1977 and 2007. SOURCE: Milligan and Wise (2011).

they did in 1977. If we add up such differences from age 55 to age 69, men in this age group worked on average 3.7 fewer years in 2007 than in 1977 (8.3 versus 12.0 years, a decline of 31 percent). Or, if at each mortality rate, men in 2007 worked as much as men in 1977, employment in the 55-69 age range would have been approximately 45 percent greater than it was. This metric suggests that there is unused capacity to work at older ages today.

Figures 5-5 and 5-6 highlight the changing relationship between mortality and employment. Mortality lends itself to these comparisons because mortality is comparable across time and across countries. Other potential measures of health status are not comparable across countries and may not be comparable across time within countries. Nonetheless, the committee also would like to explore the relationship between mortality and another

---

later, in 2007, the mortality rate was only 1.5 percent. That is to say, for the employment rate to be 50 percent in 2007, men "had to be" much healthier (by the mortality measure) than they were in 1977.

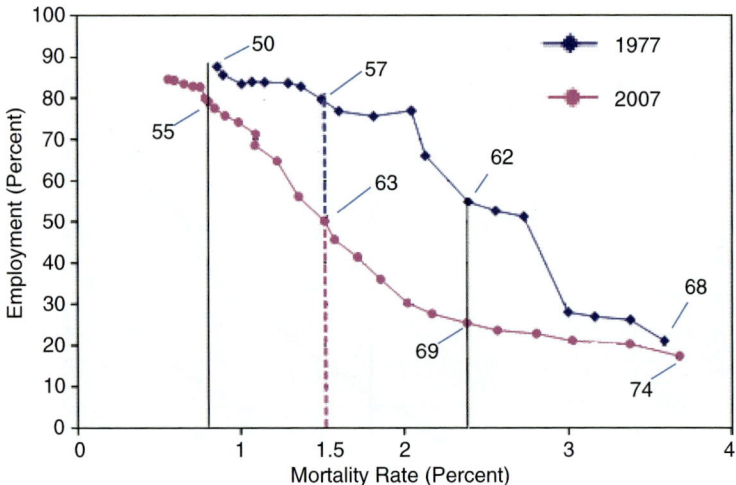

FIGURE 5-6 Employment by mortality for men, 1977 and 2007. SOURCE: Milligan and Wise (2011).

commonly used summary measure of health status, self-assessed health (SAH) status. These two measures are compared in several ways. The committee first compares SAH and future mortality in the United States. Second, it compares mortality-equivalent ages over time with SAH-equivalent ages over time. Third, it considers the time trend relationship between mortality and SAH within countries and combines the comparisons to estimate the cross-country relationship between the change in mortality over time and the comparable change in SAH over the same time period.

Self-Assessed Health and Future Mortality in the United States

Data from the U.S. Health and Retirement Study (HRS) can be used to illustrate the relationship between SAH and mortality. Table 5-1 shows, for each of five SAH categories in 1992, the proportion of men and women who were deceased by 1996, 2002, and 2008. These HRS data clearly indicate that SAH in 1992 was strongly predictive of subsequent mortality. For example, of men who reported that they were in excellent health in 1992, 11.4 percent were deceased by 2008. On the other hand, of men who reported that they were in poor health in 1992, 57.9 percent were deceased by 2008.

TABLE 5-1 Percent of Initial (1992) HRS Respondents Deceased by 1996, 2002, and 2008, by Self-Reported Health Status in 1992

	Self-Reported Health Status in 1992				
	Excellent	Very Good	Good	Fair	Poor
Men					
1996	1.0	1.5	2.1	4.3	10.8
2002	5.8	7.2	13.3	22.1	36.9
2008	11.4	15.6	25.8	36.5	57.9
Women					
1996	0.4	0.8	0.8	2.1	4.2
2002	2.6	5.4	7.1	15.2	24.4
2008	6.4	10.3	15.2	28.8	36.8

SOURCE: Milligan and Wise (2011).

Mortality-Equivalent Ages versus SAH-Equivalent Ages

"Mortality-equivalent ages" are defined as the ages at which the mortality rate was the same in different years. "SAH-equivalent ages" are defined similarly but are based on self-assessed health rather than mortality. Figure 5-7, which compares these two measures, shows that a person aged 67 in 2007 had about the same mortality rate as a person aged 60 in 1977,

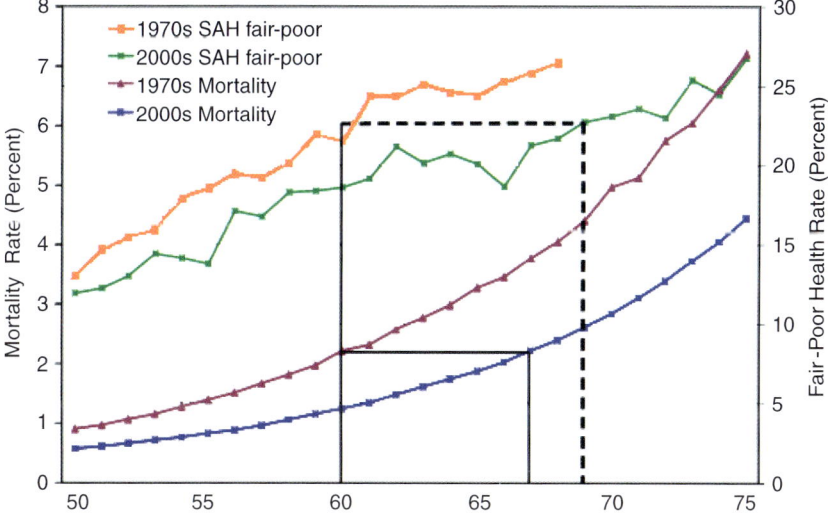

FIGURE 5-7 Mortality and self-assessed health, 1970s and 2000s. SOURCE: Milligan and Wise (2011).

a difference of 7 years. The figure also shows that men who were 69 in the 2000s had about the same SAH as men who were 9 years younger (age 60) in the 1970s. Thus in this example there was a greater difference in age-equivalent SAH than in age-equivalent mortality (about 9 versus 7 years).

Cross-Country Comparisons of Change in Mortality and Change in SAH

Figure 5-8 summarizes the SAH-mortality relationship across 11 countries for which both series are available over a sufficient time period. It compares the percent change in "fair or poor" health with the percent change in mortality. For each country, the time period spans the year of the first SAH observation to the year of the last SAH observation. For example, the period for the Netherlands is 1983 to 2008, and the percent changes in SAH and in mortality are changes between the 1983 and 2008 values. For the nine countries that report the proportion in fair or poor health, there is a close relationship between the change in mortality and the change in SAH.[4] This suggests a fairly tight within-country relationship between improvements in mortality and improvements in SAH, providing a link between the committee's earlier mortality analysis and one commonly used health measure. The committee emphasizes, however, that the level of SAH varies greatly from country to country, consistent with substantial country-specific SAH response effects.

Potential for Work in the United States

Available estimates of the future workforce, such as those produced by the BLS, assume a healthy population and do not account for a number of factors that are known to be associated with participation in the workforce, including functional impairment (Toossi, 2009). An alternative approach is to estimate the potential for work at older ages. The committee considers two such approaches here.

Cutler, Meara, and Richards-Shubik (2011) estimate the relationship between labor force participation on the one hand and demographic and health characteristics on the other for persons aged 62-64. Then they use these estimates to simulate the potential labor force participation for persons aged 65-69, which they call "capacity for work." Results for men with a high school degree or less and for men with any college are shown in Figure 5-9. The observed labor force participation, which is affected by Medicare eligibility and Social Security provisions, is compared with the

---

[4]The data points for France and the United Kingdom use different measures of health; the latter reports the percent in bad health and the former reports the average of a 10-point scale of health status.

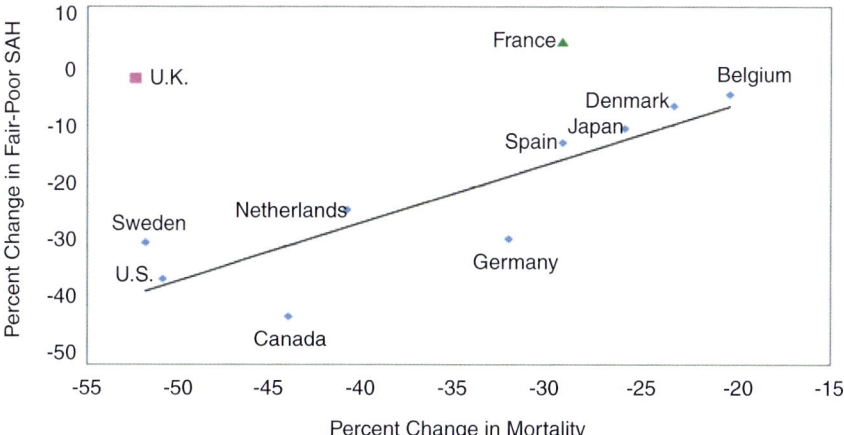

FIGURE 5-8 Percent change in "fair-poor" health and in mortality, men aged 60-64 in 11 countries. SOURCE: Milligan and Wise (2011).

simulated participation, which does not account for the effect of Medicare or Social Security provisions on retirement. For both education groups the simulated labor force participation is substantially higher than the observed rate—53 versus 35 percent for the high school or less group and 60 versus 38 percent for the any-college group. In other words, the capacity to work

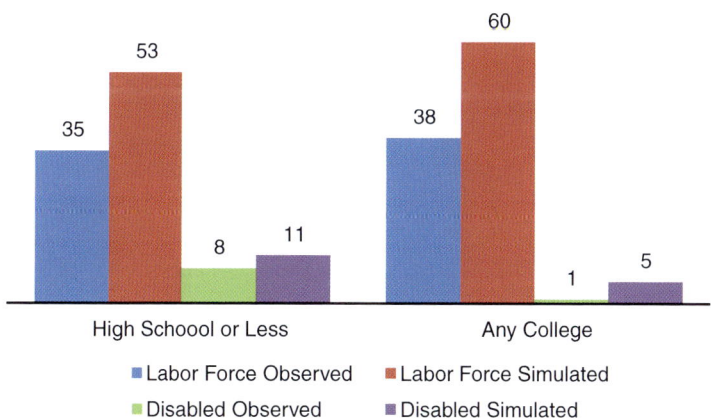

FIGURE 5-9 Labor force participation and disability rates for men aged 65-69, by education, 2000-2003. SOURCES: Based on data from the National Center for Health Statistics multiple-cause-of-death file; public-use 2000 sample census data from the U.S. Census Bureau; and data from the Medical Expenditure Panel Survey; see Cutler, Meara, and Richards-Shubik (2011) for further details.

was 51 percent greater than the actual level for high school graduates and 58 percent greater than the actual level for those with any college education. The simulated proportion for disability is also higher than the observed proportion, but the difference is very small relative to the difference in labor force participation.

A second approach, which builds on the Cutler, Meara, and Richards-Shubik analysis, was produced by a team of researchers commissioned by the committee (Rehkopf, Adler, and Rowe, 2011). The approach first considers the proportion of the population working with the proportion not working but with different levels of functional impairment. Figure 5-10 shows the distributions of men and women who are (1) working, (2) not working and with major impairment, (3) not working and with minor impairment, and (4) not working and with no impairment. These proportions are based on the average of data from nine waves of the HRS. Major impairment is defined as having limitation in one or more activities of daily living (ADL) or instrumental activities of daily living (IADL). Minor impairment is defined as not being able to do one of the following: walk several blocks, climb a flight of stairs, sit for 2 hours, and stoop, kneel, or crouch (Crimmins and Beltrán-Sánchez, 2011). As expected, the proportion of persons working is lower at older ages, and the proportion of persons with major or minor impairment is greater at older ages. However, with advancing age, large fractions of the population who are not working have

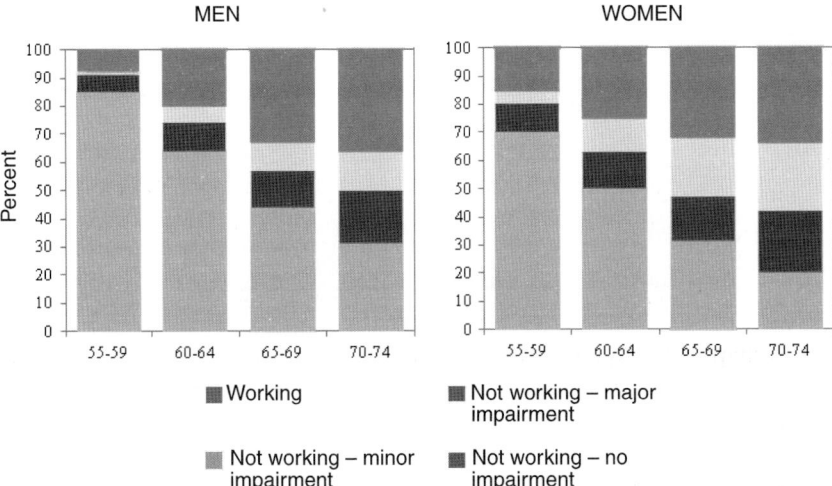

FIGURE 5-10 Percent of older population working and not working, by age and sex, composite HRS data for 1992 to 2008. SOURCE: Rehkopf, Adler, and Rowe (2011).

no impairment. For example, among men aged 65-69 who are not working, more than half have no impairment. Even at ages 70-74, half of men not working have no impairment. These data suggest that the capacity to work is substantially greater than the proportion actually working at older ages. Furthermore, while mild disability increases the likelihood of not working, many individuals with such impairments are able to continue in the workforce.

The Rehkopf, Adler, and Rowe study also made predictions of the potential workforce aged 20-74 between now and 2050, based on an evaluation of the impact of various independent predictor variables (race, ethnicity, education, father's and mother's level of education, occupation, major impairment, minor impairment, obesity, diabetes, cancer, heart disease, and stroke) on current work status using HRS data, and on projected labor force data described in Appendix A. The study considered three different assumptions about the change in disability rates in coming years: a 1 percent annual increase, no change, and a 1 percent annual decrease. Assuming no change in disability, the study forecasts a slight decrease from the current 91 percent capacity to work to 89 percent capacity to work in 2050 among the population aged 20-74. This decline reflects changes in the projected composition of the population with respect to the predictor variables. Assuming a 1 percent annual decrease in disability, the study finds a modest rise in the capacity to work over the next four decades. Only under the assumption of a 1 percent annual increase in disability is there a significant decline in the potential workforce.

In short, the evidence suggests that there is substantial potential for increased labor force participation at older ages. There has been a large decline in death rates over the past three or four decades and a corresponding improvement in self-assessed health. There has been a substantial increase in mortality-equivalent ages. For example, a person aged 67 in 2007 had about the same mortality rate as a person aged 60 in 1977. In addition, estimates of the capacity for work at older ages suggest that the potential for work is much larger that the proportion of persons actually working.

FACILITATING LONGER WORKING LIVES

Perhaps the two most important ways to facilitate longer working lives are (1) to eliminate the incentives in Social Security and private pension plans that encourage early retirement and penalize work at older ages and (2) to abandon the "fixed number of jobs" view of the labor market that has served as a rationale for maintaining program provisions that encourage older persons to leave the labor force. These issues are addressed in turn. The chapter then turns to analysis based on defined benefit (DB) plans in the United States, which have the same incentives as the social security program incentives in many countries. It then considers other issues that may promote or inhibit work at older ages.

Effect of Social Security Plan Provisions on the Incentive to Retire

Very strong evidence on the effect of pension plans on retirement is provided by cross-country comparisons of social security programs, which often have incentives like those inherent in employer-provided DB pension plans. The evidence presented is based on a coordinated set of studies conducted by analysts in each of the 12 countries in the International Social Security Project (e.g., Gruber and Wise, 1999 and 2007).

To assess the incentives for early retirement in each country's program, a measure of these incentives called the "implicit social security tax" was developed. It summarizes the extent to which earnings from working one additional year (rather than retiring) are offset by the forgone pension benefit. To understand this measure, one might think of wage compensation from working an additional year as having two components. The first is earnings from wages, and the second is the increase in the expected present discounted value of future social security benefits. One might normally expect this difference to be positive, or at least not negative. In other words, if someone works one additional year and thereby receives one less year of benefits, it might be expected that when benefits begin one year later, they are increased sufficiently to offset the fact that they are received for one less year. For example, if the typical U.S. worker does not claim Social Security benefits at the earliest possible age (62) and instead works another year, benefits in subsequent years are increased by 6.7 percent to account for the fact that they will be paid for one less year.

In most of the countries covered by the International Social Security Project, however, benefit accrual is negative. This is due in large part to the fact that benefits are not increased sufficiently when benefit receipt is postponed, i.e., benefits are not actuarially fair. Therefore, a worker's gain in extra wage earnings is partially, or even largely, offset by a loss in eventual social security benefits. The ratio of this loss to wage earnings (after tax) is called the social security implicit tax on earnings. In many countries this tax can amount to 80 percent or more at some ages.

To provide a simple summary of country-specific incentives for early retirement, the implicit tax rates on continued work are summed from age 55 or from the early retirement age—when a person initially is eligible for social security benefits—through age 69. This measure is called the "tax force to retire" (Gruber and Wise, 1999). The relationship between the tax force to retire and the proportion of men aged 55-65 not in the labor force is shown in Figure 5-11. There is a striking correspondence between the tax force to retire and men out of the labor force (unused labor capacity).

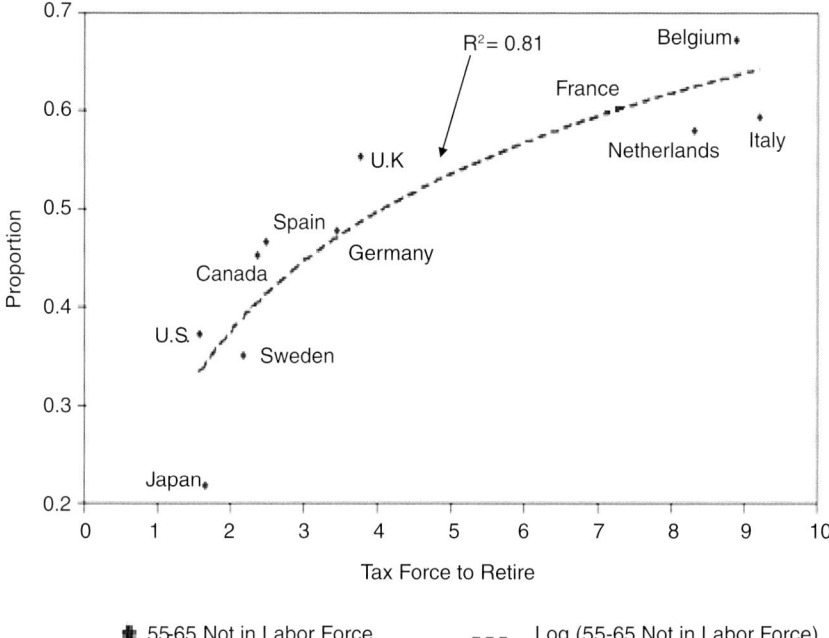

FIGURE 5-11 Tax force to retire and proportion of men aged 55-65 out of the labor force, 11 countries, circa 1995. SOURCE: Gruber, Milligan, and Wise (2009).

This suggests that social security incentives to retire are an important cause of the low labor force participation of older workers. An equally important result from this early project work is that when thinking about incentives to retire, it is critical to include disability insurance and special unemployment insurance programs as well as social security programs per se, because disability and special unemployment programs often serve as early retirement programs before the social security early retirement age.

The "Fixed Number of Jobs" View of the Labor Market

The original impetus for plan provisions that encouraged older persons to leave the labor force is unclear. It is now frequently claimed that such provisions were designed to generate more jobs for younger people, the assumption being that having fewer older persons in the labor force would translate into more opportunities for the young. This reasoning is also used against efforts to reduce or eliminate incentives for older workers to leave the labor force, by arguing that an increase in labor force participation at older ages would reduce employment among younger people. Here the committee refers to this claim as the "fixed number of jobs" assumption,[5] drawing on the International Social Security Project for evidence on whether more work by older people reduces job opportunities for younger people.

> At first glance, it seems clear that the number of jobs in economies is not fixed. "The flow of women into the labor force in the past few decades has increased the size of the labor force enormously in many countries. For example, the number of women in the labor force in the United Stated increased by almost 48 million between 1960 and 2007, from about 34 to 46 percent of the labor force. But the employment rate of men changed little as the proportion of women employed increased." (Gruber, Milligan, and Wise, 2009, p. 7)

The International Social Security Project considered several different ways of assessing the relationship between the employment of the old and the young. The various estimation methods yielded very consistent results and found no evidence that lowering employment among older people would generate more employment opportunities for younger people. Further, there was no indication that an increase in the employment rate for older people reduces employment opportunities for younger people. For example, Figure 5-12 is the same as Figure 5-11, except that it also shows the unemployment rate of youth aged 20-24 (based on data for an approximately 15-year period centered on 1995).

If the incentives that reduced the share of older people in the labor force were to increase employment opportunities for younger people, it seems likely that the tax force to retire would be related to the employment rate of younger people. That is, a greater tax force to retire should correlate with lower youth unemployment. In fact, however, there is a positive relationship between the tax force to retire and the unemployment of young men across countries. The greater the tax force to retire, the greater is youth unemployment. Further, a greater tax force to retire is associated with a lower youth employment rate. These findings offer no evidence to support the proposition that encouraging older people to leave the labor force frees up jobs for younger people.

A second way to assess the relationship between the employment of the old and the young is to consider within-country "natural experiment" estimates of this relationship. In some cases, one can compare employment trends for younger and older workers that preceded a social security reform with trends after the reform and assess (1) the impact of the reform on the

---

[5]This is often referred to by economists as the "lump of labor" theory. It was termed the "boxed economy" view in the International Social Security Project. Taken literally, this theory posits that if one additional older worker is employed, one younger worker has to be displaced. This implies that economies are boxed and that the size of the box cannot change.

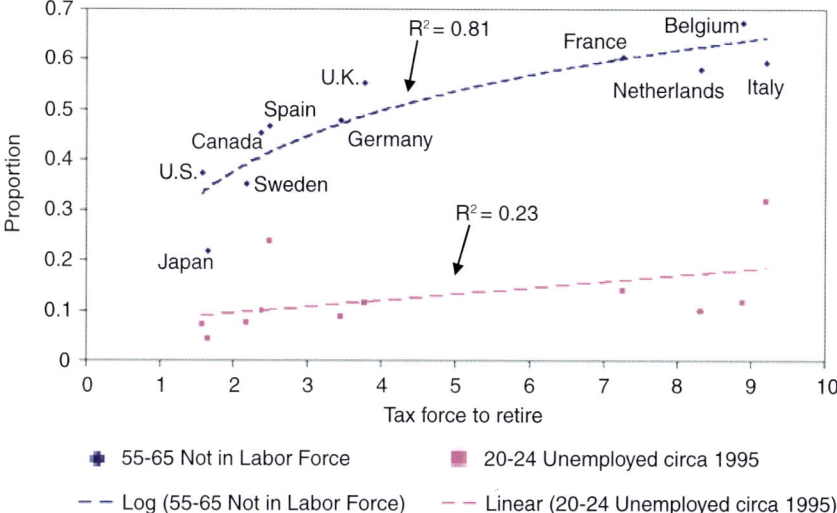

FIGURE 5-12 Tax force to retire, proportion of men aged 55-65 out of the labor force and proportion of youth aged 20-24 unemployed, circa 1995. SOURCE: Gruber, Milligan, and Wise (2009).

labor force behavior of older workers and (2) the relationship between the impact on older workers and the impact on younger workers.

A reform in Denmark provides a clear example (see Figure 5-13). In 1979, the Danish government introduced the Post-Employment Wage program, a labor market policy program intended to redistribute physically demanding jobs from older workers to unemployed younger workers. Before this reform, the youth employment rate had been rising while the youth unemployment rate changed little since 1975. Hence it seems unlikely that the reform was precipitated by a decline in the employment rate or an increase in the youth unemployment rate. Between 1978 and 1983 the employment rate for men aged 61-65 decreased by nearly 23 percentage points, a drop of 35 percent. During the same time period the employment rate for people aged 20-24 decreased by about 4 percentage points and the youth unemployment rate increased by about 4 percentage points. This natural experiment belies the fixed number of jobs proposition.[6]

---

[6]This example does not specifically address the issue of the business cycle, which may or may not have had an impact on the results. The study does, however, discuss endogeneity issues and notes that "economic shocks to the economy are likely to induce parallel movements in both the employment of the old and the employment of the young. [The study sought] to evaluate the effect of precipitating events that seek to induce older persons to leave the labor force, without a contemporaneous influence on the employment of the young (unlike macro economic shocks that tend to affect both simultaneously)" (Gruber, Milligan, and Wise, 2009, p. 23).

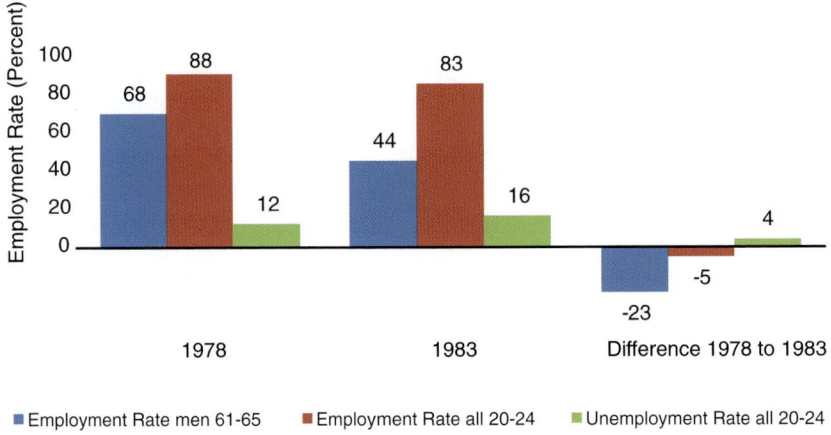

FIGURE 5-13 Response to the 1979 Post-Employment Wage reform in Denmark.
SOURCE: Gruber, Milligan, and Wise (2009).

Gruber, Milligan, and Wise (2009) cite similar natural experiments for other countries that reveal the same thing. Several additional methods have been used to assess the relationship between the employment of the young and the old. In short, natural experiments and other methods of analysis all lead to the same conclusion and "provide no support for the boxed economy proposition. Indeed, the weight of the evidence suggests that increasing the employment of older persons provides more job opportunities for younger persons and reduces the unemployment rate of younger persons." (Gruber, Milligan, and Wise, 2009, p. 64). The finding is consistent with earlier work showing that older and younger workers are actually complements, not substitutes (Levine and Mitchell, 1988).

Private DB Pension Plans Offer Large Incentive Effects to Retire Early

The social security retirement incentives described above result from the way in which the social security DB is determined in each country. Employer-provided DB pension plans typically have similar retirement incentives. DB pension plans are still common in the United States and are particularly important for state and local government employees, even as the proportion of employees covered by personal retirement plans such as 401(k) plans is rising rapidly. DB plans are also common in Canada and in the United Kingdom, and they underpin the employer-based system in the Netherlands. Thus, in some countries the incentive effects inherent in these plans can also have a large effect on labor force participation (Stock and Wise, 1990a and 1990b; Gustman and Steinmeier, 2002).

Just as for social security incentives, the key issue is this: If the receipt of benefits is delayed for a year, are benefits increased enough to offset their receipt for one less year? Is the benefit formula actuarially fair? Under the typical employer-provided DB plan in the United States, the answer is no. Benefits are not increased sufficiently to offset receipt for one less year. Thus, the plans impose a large implicit tax on work, just like the implicit tax described above for social security defined benefits. Indeed, the analysis of retirement incentives inherent in employer-provided DB plans in the United States led to the international comparison project that produced the results discussed above. The following discussion provides some information on the incentive effects of employer-provided plans. It does not attempt to draw from all the many studies that address this issue.

Until the mid-1990s, one of the important economic trends in the United States was the withdrawal of older persons from employment. This trend was surely made possible by the advent of the Social Security program and by the concurrent spread of employer-provided pension plans. Most of the pension plans were DB plans in which the benefit at retirement depended on years of service and earnings (usually those during the last years of employment).

Stock and Wise (1990a and 1990b) used company data to develop and estimate a formal model of retirement based on the option value retirement model. The model's central feature involves recognition of the significant effect on retirement of the future accrual pattern of pension benefits. A series of subsequent papers found similar behavioral responses to plan incentives among men and women and among different types of employees (see, e.g., Lumsdaine, Stock, and Wise, 1997).

Looking at social security systems in different countries was analogous to looking at the effects of different employer-sponsored pension plans (with varying provisions) in the United States. Indeed, the retirement responses to social security plan incentives to retire correspond very closely to the incentive inherent in the employer-provided DB plans.

401(k)-Like Plans Have None of These Incentive Effects

Since the early 1980s there has been a rapid conversion to 401(k) plans in the private sector and a movement away from DB plans. The data are shown in Figure 5-14. People can of course participate in more than one type of plan. The 401(k) plans and other personal accounts such as individual retirement accounts (IRAs) have none of the incentive effects of DB plans and in particular none of the early retirement incentives inherent in DB plans. Since DB plans had typically provided a strong inducement to retire early, it should be expected that the decline in DB plans reduced the incentive to retire early. Thus the advent of personal accounts probably was

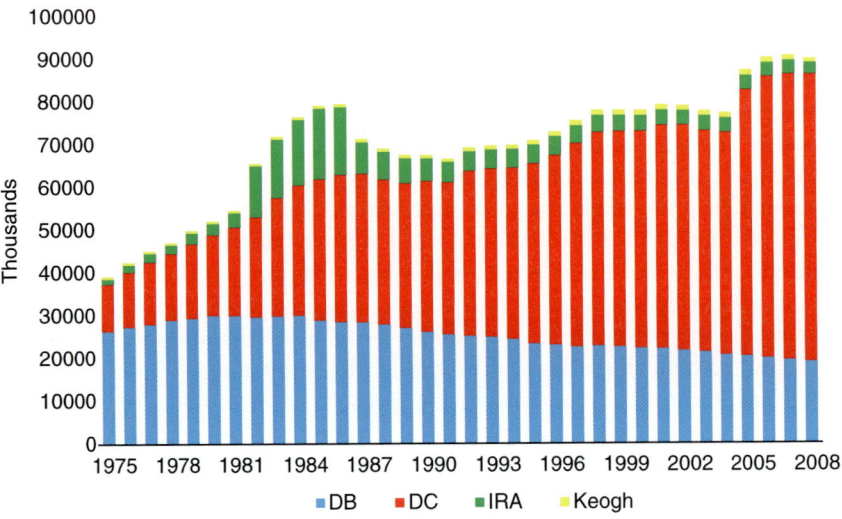

FIGURE 5-14 Pension plan participants in the private sector by plan type, 1975-2008. SOURCES: Data for defined benefit (DB) and defined contribution (DC) from Department of Labor, Form 5500; data for individual retirement accounts (IRAs) and Keogh plans from Internal Revenue Service, Statistics of Income.

one reason for the increase in the labor force participation of older workers since the mid-1990s.

State and Local DB Plans Have Strong Incentives to Retire Early

While there has been a rapid conversion to personal retirement accounts in the private sector, DB plans with strong early retirement incentives are still common among federal, state, and local employees. Figure 5-15 shows the trend in the federal (nonmilitary) sector. There is less time-series information on DB versus DC coverage for the state and local sectors. Except for a few scattered plans in higher education, there were no DC plans in state government until 1996. By 2010, 13 states offered their employees a DC plan (typically a secondary plan). Recently, Michigan and Alaska required all new employees to participate solely in a DC plan, but in these states the primary plan for earlier hires is still DB.

The best state and local data are from the BLS compensation surveys. The 2010 survey of state and local governments found that 90 percent offered retirement benefits, with 85 percent participating; that 84 percent offered a DB plan, with 79 percent participating; that 29 percent offered a DC plan, with 17 percent participating; and that most persons who were offered a DC plan were also offered a DB plan.

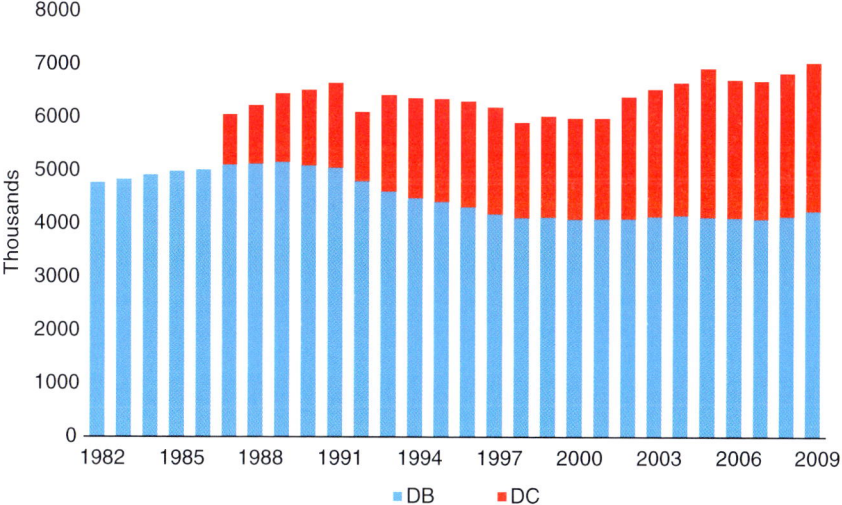

FIGURE 5-15 Pension plan participants in the federal sector, by plan type, 1982-2009. SOURCE: Employee Benefit Research Institute, *Databook on Employee Benefits*, various years.

Reducing the Cost of Employing Older Workers

It is not well known that older workers in the United States face higher effective tax rates than younger workers. For instance, the 15.3 percent Social Security and Medicare payroll tax is often a pure tax on work for those aged 60 and over (Goda, Shoven, and Slavov, 2011). That is, while younger workers accrue additional Social Security benefits from the payroll taxes they pay, older workers have often already worked the 35 years that count toward Social Security benefits. Depending on their remuneration, older workers may earn no incremental retirement benefits or Medicare benefits for continuing in the workforce. The employer and employee halves of the payroll tax combine to create a 15.3 percent wedge between wages and the worker output.

Many ways have been proposed to decrease the implicit tax on work for older workers (see, e.g., Butrica et al, 2006; Goda, Shoven, and Slavov, 2009; Kotlikoff and Wise, 1988). This report does not evaluate these options but does present two illustrative examples. One way to lessen the effect would be to create a new category of worker: "paid up." After 35 or 40 years of covered work experience, the payroll tax would be eliminated. Such workers would be paid up. One principle would be that every year of earnings either counts towards Social Security benefits or is not subject to the payroll tax. Removing a 15 percent wedge between the employer's cost of employment and the employee's net wage would be equivalent to an 18 percent increase in net pay.[7]

For many workers aged 65 and over there is an even larger implicit tax. If they work for an employer with an employee health insurance benefit and more than 20 employees, then Medicare steps aside and lets the employer-sponsored health plan cover the worker. This policy is called Medicare as a secondary payer. Depending on the incidence of the employer-sponsored health insurance, it is likely that employees pay for health insurance even though they are otherwise eligible for Medicare. This creates another large gap between the employer's cost of employing an older worker and the employee's net wage. This wedge varies by age, gender, wage, and other factors and can easily average 30 percent (Goda, Shoven, and Slavov, 2007). In combination with the payroll tax, the total wedge from these two sources can approximate 45 percent. An alternative policy would be to grant Medicare benefits to workers aged 65 and over whether their employer has a health plan or not. This policy could be termed Medicare as a primary payer. Eliminating the entire 45 percent wedge would increase net wages by over 80 percent.

Retiree Health Benefits

The substantial connection between health insurance and employment may prompt many U.S. workers to delay retirement until they are eligible for Medicare at age 65. Some employers provide health insurance to retired workers, and those who can receive such insurance may not need to wait until age 65 to retire with group health coverage. Nyce et al. (2011) investigated the relationship between retiree health insurance and early retirement using data from 64 diverse company clients of Towers Watson, a prominent benefits consulting firm. They found that retiree health coverage has a strong effect on retirement. For example, a generous employer contribution of 50 percent or more lowered the number of person-years worked between ages 56 and 64 by 9.6 percent compared to those with no coverage. This question may be particularly important in light of the health reforms enacted in 2010, which if implemented will weaken the connection between employment and health insurance by making group coverage available to all regardless of work status.

---

[7] It should be noted that while a policy involving paid-up workers could help to raise labor force participation among older persons, it might have a deleterious effect on the imbalance in the Social Security trust fund. A similar concern could arise with respect to the idea of Medicare as a primary payer.

Gradual Retirement

An important way to facilitate longer working lives is to adopt policies and practices that allow workers (and employers) greater flexibility with respect to hours worked and give people more control over job responsibilities and demands as they age. There is substantial anecdotal evidence that many older workers would prefer to work half-time, for example. As noted earlier in this chapter, gradual retirement in the United States is becoming more common. Older workers are more likely than younger workers to work part-time, and the proportion of older workers employed part-time increases with age. Sixty percent of both men and women who had left full-time employment after age 50 by 2008 had moved to a "bridge" job, with more than half of such jobs being part-time (Quinn, Cahill, and Giandrea, 2011). Many of the bridge jobs pay less than the earlier full-time jobs.

Related to this discussion is the need to consider and promote training, retraining, and continuing education for older workers. Some studies of demand and prevalence in these areas are under way, but the empirical basis for understanding how common and effective such measures have been is still lacking. One of the committee's research recommendations in Chapter 10 encourages data collection and analysis of the facilitation of work at older ages.

MACRO IMPLICATIONS OF LONGER WORKING LIVES

The changing demographic environment over the past five decades is on the one hand an achievement and on the other a problem. Chapter 3 explained that mortality rates have declined and life expectancy has increased substantially in industrialized countries. This is the achievement. The problem is that falling birth rates and fewer young people, combined with increased longevity, mean that the ratio of old to young is rising. An increasing number of older people means that health care costs will rise not only because of sheer numbers but also because technology will likely lead to improved and probably more expensive treatment. And while the cost of public pensions rises, there is the prospect of fewer persons in the labor force to pay for the rising pension and health care costs.

How might the increasing imbalance between the rising proportion of older people and the declining proportion of young people be accommodated? Part of the solution would be to leverage the gains in longevity by increasing the employment rate of older people. This would increase the number of people in the workforce and lower the number of retirees that workers help support.

But as noted earlier, until the mid-1990s the trend was just the opposite. The employment rate for older persons in the United States was dropping, which made it increasingly difficult for the labor force to support those who had retired. In the United States, the median number of years in retirement for men increased nearly 50 percent between 1965 and 2003, from 13 years to almost 19 years. Roughly half of these additional years were related to gains in life expectancy and the other half to earlier retirement (Goda, Shoven, and Slavov, 2009). In other industrialized countries, the trend has been more extreme. Figure 5-16 shows the percent increase in life expectancy at age 65 together with the percent decline in the labor force participation of men aged 60-64 in the 12 countries participating in the International Social Security Project. In all of the countries life expectancy has increased and in all of the countries labor force participation has declined, although there is substantial variation across countries.

What is the gain from prolonged labor force participation? An increase in the labor force participation of older persons will increase production (gross domestic product). Increased production will increase tax revenues, which should in turn increase available funding for social security and health care. In addition, personal savings may increase with longer working lives. This would essentially happen by default with 401(k)-like personal retirement accounts. Because a large portion of private saving is through personal retirement accounts, this effect may offset the possibility that some persons would save less because they anticipated the need to support fewer retirement years. In the United States, an increasingly large proportion of resources has been going to health care and pensions for older persons. If the resources of the country are to advance in future years, the education of the current young is of critical importance. If the working lives of older people lengthen, not only will there be more resources to pay Social Security

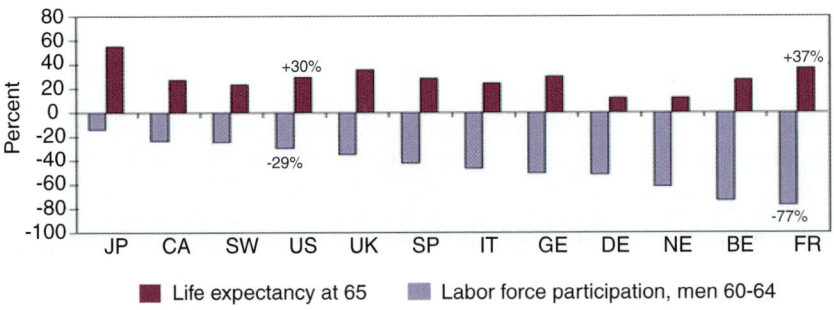

FIGURE 5-16 Increase in life expectancy and decline in labor force participation in 12 countries, 1960s to early 2000s. JP-Japan; CA-Canada; SW-Sweden; US-United States; UK-United Kingdom; SP-Spain; IT-Italy; GE-Germany; DE-Denmark; NE-Netherlands; BE-Belgium; FR-France. SOURCE: Data compiled as part of the National Bureau of Economic Research International Social Security Project.

and health care costs, but also more resources will be freed up to pay for the education of the young.

Of course, there may be trade-offs for later retirement ages. Data from the Health and Retirement Study show that roughly one-fourth of workers aged 60-61 report a health condition that limits their work capability. Raising the early retirement age would delay benefit eligibility and might lead older people with job-limiting health conditions to seek disability insurance rather than waiting to claim retirement. Raising the full retirement age would reduce retirement benefits for people who retire early and might generate a financial incentive to seek disability insurance benefits, which are not reduced (Government Accountability Office, 2010).

Nevertheless, two key ingredients are critical to facilitating longer working lives. First, penalties on work at older ages—found in the provisions of many employer-provided DB pension plans and in many national social security programs—that encourage older people to leave the labor force would have to be eliminated. In the United States these provisions have been reduced by the conversion to 401(k) and other personal retirement accounts. But DB pension plans are still common for state and local employees, who typically have very generous plans with strong inducements to retire early. Second, a false rationale—the assumption of a fixed number of jobs in the economy—used to maintain provisions that encourage older people to leave employment would have to be abandoned. In addition, it will be important to understand which work arrangements, such as flexible working hours, would facilitate work by older persons and to assess the potential of employers to accommodate such arrangements.

Finally, automatic adjustment of Social Security benefits may help accommodate the force of demographic change. Many analysts have suggested that retirement ages be indexed to longevity. By 2009, 13 out of 30 OECD countries had introduced automatic links of pension benefits to life expectancy in their public pension systems (OECD, 2009). Systems in Sweden and Italy link benefits to life expectancy, the dependency ratio, and wage growth. Germany has maintained a DB system but bases benefits on a "sustainability factor." Annual benefit changes are determined by changes in gross earnings minus contributions to the pension system and by changes in the dependency ratio (Boersch-Supan, Reil-Held, and Wilke, 2007; Boersch-Supan and Ludwig, 2010). As noted elsewhere in this report, however, policies that link retirement ages (particularly the full retirement age) to overall life expectancy might lower benefits disproportionately for those with a shorter life expectancy, a less than desirable distributional effect.

6

Aging, Productivity, and Innovation

BACKGROUND

One of the important issues raised by the aging society is its impact on productivity, adaptation, and innovation. Improvements in productivity play a central role in the growth of long-run living standards, and an important aspect of a society is its ability to innovate and adapt to changing conditions. It is worth remembering that small changes in productivity growth will lead to large improvements in living standards over time.

There has been relatively little research on the impact of a changing age structure on overall economic productivity. There are many ways in which changes in the age distribution can affect productivity. For example, the performance of certain tasks may differ over the life cycle. There is substantial research on different ages in the psychology literature. But actual productivity is more complicated than the undertaking of simple tasks, and experience, work skills, health status, job turnover, and other more subtle factors also have a major impact on productivity. The net effect, as best as the committee can judge from the literature, is that there is likely to be little net effect of changes in the age distribution on productivity in the United States over the next two decades.

Productivity growth is commonly measured as the growth of output per unit of input, either per unit of labor input or per unit of all factors combined. Analyses of productivity growth generally separate the determinants of labor productivity growth into those generated by (1) increases in the quantity and quality of inputs combined with labor and (2) technological change, either new or improved products or improved processes of production.

The first factor—increases in productivity due to higher inputs—would include the improved education, training, and skill acquisition of labor as well as higher quality and quantity of complementary factors such as capital and resources. For example, increased levels of education of the workforce improve the quality of labor inputs and thereby increase output per hour worked. Changes in the quantity of inputs would be the first important channel through which an aging population could change productivity. As the workforce ages, it becomes more experienced, and greater experience is generally associated with higher earnings and productivity. But an aging workforce might also experience deterioration in the relevant skills if job requirements change over time or if people's skills decline. Some believe, for example, that increased penetration of information technologies into the workplace might place older workers at a disadvantage. This chapter will review below the evidence on how these factors interact in the workplace.

The second factor in productivity growth involves ingredients other than increases of inputs. Called "technological advance," it also includes advances in knowledge and organization and has a completely different mechanism. Over the long run, technological advance arises from several channels: the generation and diffusion of new scientific, technological, and engineering knowledge and improvements in production processes and social overhead capital. For example, the vast improvements in productivity in computation arose from a long line of technological developments, from transistors to improved communications to programmable software. Innovations in organizational structure and management practices and improved political and legal environments have also fostered significant productivity gains. While technological advance and other changes have played a key role in productivity growth, their rate and direction have varied greatly from decade to decade, and the pattern of change is not well understood.

Studies of productivity growth and technological change emphasize that progress does not typically occur through a grand leap by a single ingenious inventor. Rather, improvements in products and processes are typically the result of many small and unspectacular steps. They result from the application of basic research and engineering, from learning by doing, and from suggestions by workers on the production line.

Clearly, the processes involved in increasing productivity involve both very local forces, such as the skills of individual workers, and more global trends in new and improved technologies and processes. Moreover, economic studies indicate that the second factor—technological advance—is the major contributor to long-run growth in productivity. Depending on the time, place, and approach, studies indicate that anywhere from half to virtually all of the growth in output per hour worked or per capita income is due to advances in knowledge, and that the balance is due to increases in capital and other inputs per unit of labor.

RESEARCH ON THE IMPACTS OF AGING AT THE INDIVIDUAL LEVEL

There is a substantial literature on behavioral measures of productivity or proxies for it over the life cycle. Studies include psychometric ones (such as ones that measure verbal or quantitative reasoning), ratings (such as those of supervisors), productivity measures (such as in piece rates or baseball scores), and statistical studies at the company level. Useful surveys are those by Prskawetz and Lindh (2006) and Skirbekk (2004).

On the whole, the literature on individual productivity measures shows great diversity across age, individuals, and measures. As one of the pioneers in the field, Salthouse (1991) found that the relationship between age and cognition varies considerably across different cognitive tests.

Many psychometric measures show a clear relationship to age. Verhaegen and Salthouse (1997) provide a meta-analysis of cognitive studies (p. 246). They compare the performance of individuals over and under 50 years of age and conclude as follows:

> [M]eta-analyses of correlations between age and different measures of cognition revealed that the age relations in this literature are somewhat stronger with measures of speed than with measures of reasoning, spatial abilities, and working and episodic memory and that primary memory has a smaller age relation than do the latter variables.

Avolio and Waldman (1994) examine a series of studies that measure work-related skills using the General Aptitude Test Battery (GATB) for more than 25,000 workers from 16 to 74 years old. They conclude that age accounted for a relatively small percentage of the variance in ability test scores once experience, education, and occupational type were controlled. Differences in performance across age groups were relatively small until at least age 65. However, unlike the earnings data reviewed below, job experience has little value in predicting the maintenance of abilities over the long run except for complex jobs.

Literature using other metrics for individual productivity also shows divergent results by age and metric. One survey concludes that supervisors' ratings typically do not find any clear systematic relationship between age and productivity. The evidence on productivity as measured by piece rates is mixed.

An important new approach is cross-sectional employer-employee matched data. These studies also show a mixed pattern, with many studies estimating peak productivity at around 40 years of age, while a few find peak productivity at older ages. Case studies in the United States and Germany shed more light on the age-productivity relation. Kotlikoff and Wise (1989) found that the productivity of salespeople in a large insurance company, measured by the value of contracts sold, increases with age. Boersch-Supan, Duezguen, and Weiss (2008) and Boersch-Supan and Weiss (2011) assembled a large data set on production workers in a German car manufacturing company over many years and show a similar effect. They measure productivity by the absence of errors in a well-defined production process. They find that, while the number of small errors is larger among older workers, major errors are more frequent among younger ones. Their measure of productivity finds that older workers have higher productivity.

Although the literature on productivity and behavior at the individual level provides weighty evidence on the impact of aging on many individual attributes, we need to be cautious about the application of those attributes to aggregate productivity. Many of the studies are cross-sectional and do not take into account changes in occupation or, in labor market studies, attrition.

Additionally, the determinants of individual productivity are extremely complex and are unlikely to be captured in most metrics. For example, a typical cross-sectional study of earnings can explain a small fraction of the dispersion on the basis of personal attributes such as intelligence. Moreover, while it is true in a few areas that reasonable output metrics have been developed (such as for athletes), we know that in other areas the measures have often proven highly unreliable and even systemically dangerous (such as the compensation metrics used in many financial firms).

Furthermore, the important skill sets, and the difficulties in accurately measuring them, will change over the life cycle as workers move from being unskilled workers at fast food stores in summer jobs, to entry-level technicians, to middle and upper management positions. Given the multitude of attributes and vast number of different jobs, it has proven very difficult to make an accurate measure of the economic value of an individual's attributes and the changes in those over time due to aging.

A final reason to discount metrics on individual attributes is that work increasingly takes place in teams. Teams are often composed of individuals with different backgrounds and experiences, and it is difficult to separate the contribution of individuals. So while we might focus on the hitting scores of star baseball players, it is worth considering how well nine players would perform in the absence of (generally older) coaches, trainers, surgeons, and owners. In an economy, it is generally the bundle or teams that are productive, not the individuals.

For this reason, the committee tends to prefer market-based measures to estimate the impact of aging on productivity, either measures based on market earnings or ones based on aggregate measures of productivity.

AGING AND THE ECONOMICS OF INNOVATION AND INVENTION

The first important question involves the impact of changes in the age distribution of the population on a society's innovation and invention. An important aspect of new knowledge is that it is a public good, a process in which new technologies generated anywhere can potentially spread and be used by all, young and old, rich and poor, at home and abroad. Hence the stock of useful and productive knowledge should be seen in the context of the global stock rather than that of an individual person or country. If other countries take up more of the innovational activities that were over the last century led by the United States and other current high-income countries, the overall trend in income and productivity growth might well continue to grow rapidly. So a first important point is that it is global inventive and innovative activity that over the coming decades will influence long-run U.S. productivity and income growth. Countries are not technological islands in an increasingly globalized world. As countries grow and increase their inventive activity in an increasingly networked world, the United States will benefit from the inventiveness outside its borders (Jones and Romer, 2010).

While long-run productivity growth is likely to be largely determined by global trends in frontier technologies, national characteristics are critical for diffusion and adoption of best-practice technologies and for actual levels of productivity. Studies of diffusion show that best-practice knowledge and techniques diffuse more slowly across national borders than within nations. The rate of adoption depends on many non-age-related factors, such as openness to trade and capital flows; competitiveness of domestic market structures; profitability; and regulatory structures. The major impacts of age-related factors reflect the composition of demand. For example, an aging population or one with strong demand for health services is likely not only to generate but also to adopt technologies that are in great domestic demand in this sector.

There is a substantial literature on the age distribution of producers of inventions, patents, publications, and other creative material. Historians of science have generally concluded that scientific output tends to rise steeply in the twenties and thirties, peak in the late thirties or early forties, and then trail off slowly through later years. There is some variation among disciplines, but most studies find that peak scientific productivity tends to be in the interval between ages 30 and 40 (Lehman, 1953; Simonton, 1988 and 1991).

Benjamin Jones (2010) has investigated the question of age and "great achievement" in a statistical framework using data covering more than a century. His sample is of Nobel prize winners in physics, chemistry, medicine, and economics ($N = 544$) and great technological inventors ($N = 286$). Figure 6-1 shows the age distribution for each group from his sample. In each case, the average age was 39.[1] There is considerable dispersion in the distribution.

Another important finding of Jones's study is that the average age at which invention occurred increased over the twentieth century. For recipients of Nobel prizes in physics, chemistry, and medicine, the increase in the median age has been around 2 years per century, while the increase in the mean has been 8 years. The increase has resulted from an increase in the starting age (the age at which the youngest inventors did their prize-winning work) as well as the ending age (the age at which oldest inventors did their prize-winning work). In part, the increase in the ending age is due to the longer life span over which invention occurs that comes from longer life expectancy.

From a policy perspective, one of the most important findings is a delay in the start of the creative period. Jones finds a significant delay in the onset of scientific creativity. He points to two potential factors in the delay: the increased complexity of acquiring knowledge because of the greater depth of accumulated knowledge and the longer time to a final degree (see also National Research Council, 1990 and 1998).

There is genuine concern on the part of the scientific establishment in universities as well as federal scientific agencies that the longer time for young researchers to enter their careers as productive scientists is due to institutional impediments.

Patents and Other Areas

Another measure of innovative output, and one that is generally closer to economic activity, is patents. Patents have been the subject of study as indicators of inventive output for many years (see the overview in Griliches, 1990). They have the advantage of passing some threshold of importance and nonobviousness. Their shortcoming is that they have highly variable importance and commercial value. Jones (2009) examined the characteristics of patent awardees over the twentieth century and found increases in three important measures: (1) the age at which an inventor makes the first invention; (2) a measure of specialization in patents; and (3) the size of teams. He concludes that the nature of the scientific and inventive process is becoming more complicated as more knowledge is accumulated. Additionally, the age at which applied knowledge was crystallized in the form

---

[1] Age refers to the age at which a discovery was made, as best as could be determined.

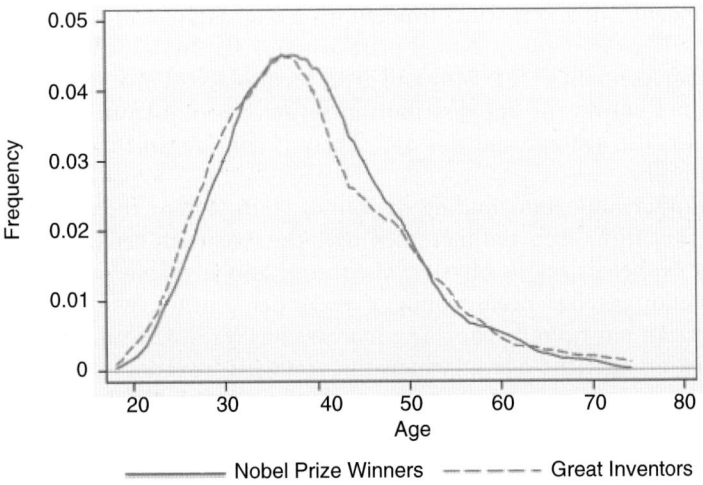

FIGURE 6-1 Age distribution of great inventors and Nobel prize winners. SOURCE: Jones (2010). Reprinted by permission.

of patents tends to be about a decade later than transformational science or great inventions.

Other studies have examined the age of artistic creation, such as for works of fine art (Galenson 2004a and 2004b). There appears to be greater dispersion in the ages of creative works than of scientific achievements. Galenson also distinguishes between conceptual innovations (done at an early age) and experimental creativity (often performed at a later age). But the basic idea about the distinctive role of the early years (from 25 to 45 years of age) emerges from these other studies as well.

Determinants Other Than Age

While age is an important determinant of invention and innovation, it explains very little about actual performance across societies. Other factors, such as education, support institutions, economic and social rewards, and religious institutions, tend to dominate the actual distribution of scientific output.

This can be illustrated by examining the distribution of Nobel prize awards in chemistry and physics over the last century. If we assume that the distribution of awards should be proportional to that of raw talent, and that raw talent should be equally distributed around the world, then we would expect that the number of prize winners should be distributed proportionally to the population (or young population) of different countries.

In reality, the proportion of prize winners born in Africa or India is lower by a factor of more than 100 than that of those born in Western Europe and North America. Moreover, the least developed countries, with 10 percent of the world's population, have not produced a single prize winner in physics or chemistry during the entire history of those prizes.

Put differently, over two-thirds of Nobel prize–winning research done since 1960 has occurred in the United States, even though the United States averaged only 5 percent of the world's population. The fact that 30 percent of U.S.-based Nobel prize winners were foreign born indicates the importance of the research environment for successful invention.

Looking forward, the key to continuing strong advances in knowledge for the United States and other countries is to increase investments in young scientists and other creative talent. The importance of the support environment is an emphatic reminder of the key role of educational and other social institutions in nurturing innovation. The United States has performed relatively poorly in recent years in K-12 education compared to other countries, according to the Organisation for Economic Co-Operation and Development (OECD) Programme for International Student Assessment. Also, most urban school districts in the United States see high school graduation rates of only 50 percent. These indicators are a reminder of the vast potential supply of scientific and innovational talents that remains untapped in the United States and the rest of the world, and of the important determinants of technological advance other than age.

PRODUCTIVITY AND THE AGE STRUCTURE OF THE POPULATION

The second important factor in the productivity of the population involves the interaction of the quality of the workforce and the distribution of the population with a given technology. As noted above, this influence would include the impact of improved education, training, skill acquisition of labor as well as higher quality and quantity of complementary factors such as capital and resources. In its discussion, the committee focuses on the impact of a workforce whose composition is changing; the reason for this focus is that the impact of the age distribution on complementary factors such as capital and resources appears to be less significant.

The basic idea is that workers have different productivities as a result of evolving skills, experience, formal and informal education, training, and personal attributes over their life cycles. In the human capital model, productivity is a function of the amount of accumulated human capital. Human capital will vary over the life span. Generally, we expect productivity to be relatively low for unskilled and inexperienced workers; to rise with education and experience and as workers find a good match between their skills and the opportunities in the workplace; and eventually to decline either as (or if) their skills decline or their specific human capital and experience depreciate.

A central issue in this context is the age distribution of productivity for the workforce. Changes in aggregate productivity arise from the interaction of the age distribution of productivity and the changing age distribution of the labor force. This can be called the "age composition effect." A plot of this effect would be analogous to the productivity curve shown in Figure 6-1, although it would look quite different. There are two alternative approaches to estimating the age composition effect. The first examines the age distribution of earnings and assumes that earnings are proportional to productivity. The second looks directly at the impact of the age distribution on aggregate productivity.

Earnings and the Changing Distribution of the Workforce

There is a vast literature on the distribution of earnings by different attributes, including age, experience, and education. A recent survey of this approach summarized the results as follows:

> Perhaps the most widely estimated regression equation in economics is Mincer's log-earnings function that relates the log of individual earnings or wages to observed measures of schooling and potential work experience. The regression has been estimated in numerous studies, employing various data sets from almost every historical period and country for which micro data are available, with remarkably robust regularities. First, workers' wage profiles are well ranked by education level; at any experience level, workers earn more, on average, as their schooling increases. Second, average wages grow at a decreasing rate until late in one's working lifetime. (Rubinstein and Weiss, 2006, p. 3)

In the simplest approach, with perfectly competitive markets, a worker's hourly earnings are equal to the value of the marginal product of an hour worked. This relationship would hold even if the worker is investing in general (non-firm-specific) human capital. Labor economists have reservations about this theory. The link between current earnings and current marginal productivity may be decoupled if there are long-term relations or contracts between the worker and the company. In some areas, for example, compensation is back-loaded to provide incentives for workers to stay with companies. Additionally, most earnings estimates exclude fringe benefits such as health care, which are an increasingly important fraction of total compensation. While labor economists generally believe that fringe benefits are a dollar-for-dollar substitute for wages, this may hold for the company and is unlikely to hold for individual workers in large companies, so examination of earnings without fringe benefits is an appropriate approach. While the earnings-marginal productivity theory has many shortcomings, it does provide a useful benchmark for purposes of estimating the impact of a changing age structure.

The examples provided here take the simplest case in which earnings are assumed to be proportional to marginal productivities.[2] This specification initially assumes no impact of changes in the distribution of the labor force on relative earnings or productivity, and this assumption will be relaxed below.

The standard earnings-age-experience model assumes that earnings are a quadratic function of age or experience. A careful review of the data indicates that this introduces inaccurate estimates in the tails of the distribution. It underestimates the growth of earnings in the early years and overestimates the decline in the later years. Since these are exactly the years that are important for present purposes, estimation of distributional effects is accordingly uncertain.

For the present purpose, the committee took estimates of the age-earnings profile for college graduates and high school graduates. The estimates are drawn from a study by Lemieux (2006) based on earlier work of Murphy and Welch (1990) and are very similar to those made by Rubinstein and Weiss (2006). The Lemieux estimates rely on 1999-2001 Current Population Survey data on hourly earnings with a dummy for education and for year. Estimates of the earnings-experience curve are shown in Figure 6-2. The shaded line is the unconstrained curve, while the other two show the results using quadratic and quartic functions of experience.

To generate estimates of the impact of a changing age distribution on productivity, the committee used the 1999-2001 age-experience curve as its age-productivity relationship in conjunction with the committee's estimates and projections of the distribution of the labor force by age (see Appendix A) for three different years, 2010, 2020, and 2030, and applied the estimates for males to all workers. This yields three different experience curves: the quadratic fits the standard quadratic function to the actual data; the quartic fit is the result of Lemieux's equation; and the actual is the unconstrained age-experience curve. These results are shown in Table 6-1 separately for college and high school graduates.

---

[2]The procedure for estimating the age composition effect assumes that the workforce has a distribution given by $\{\theta_{1,t},..., \theta_{n,t}\}$, where $\theta_{i,t}$ is the share of the labor force, employment, or population in age group i and time period t. We assume that productivity is a separable function of the share of workers in each age group and of other factors. Then we can write the aggregate production function as

$$Y_t = A_t F [H_t, K_t], H_t = \Sigma [(\theta_{i,t} L_t) w_{i,t}]$$

where L_t is total labor inputs in year t, H_t is an index of aggregate labor input, K_t is capital and other inputs, $w_{i,t}$ is average earnings of group i, and A_t is an index of technology.

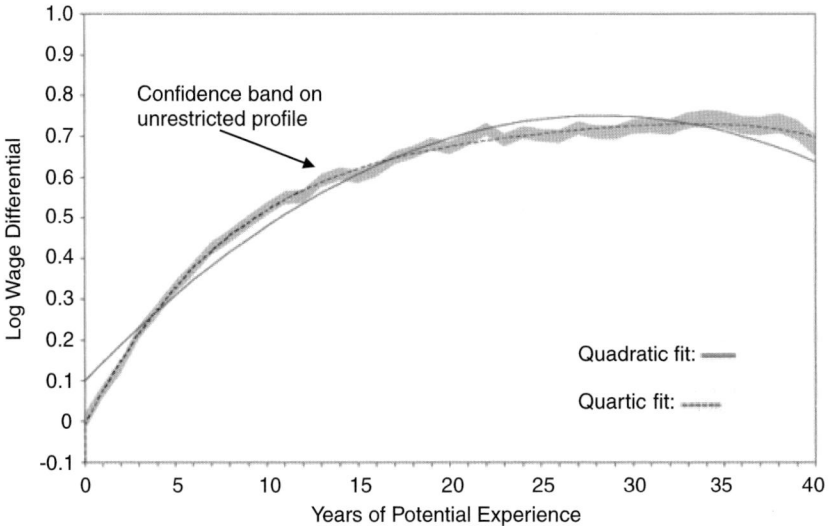

FIGURE 6-2 Distribution of earnings, by age. This figure shows the unrestricted (shaded band) as well as quadratic and quartic fit to the ln wage data for males using data from the 1999-2001 Current Population Survey. The series are estimated with a full set of education, experience, and year dummies. SOURCE: Lemieux (2006). Reprinted by permission.

Note that the earnings functions usually do not go beyond 40 years of experience (taken to be 62 years of age for college graduates and 58 years for high school graduates). Therefore, this analysis takes the distribution only through 40 years of experience, which covers between 87 and 91 percent of the distribution depending upon the year. There is some truncation bias, but this appears to make little difference to the estimates.[3]

Table 6-1 shows the calculated impact of the changing age distribution on the rate of growth of productivity over the 2010-2020 and 2020-2030 periods. The estimates suggest that the age composition effect is likely to be very small for all specifications and both periods. The largest positive number is 0.024 percentage points per year and the largest negative estimate is −0.013 percentage points per year. For reference purposes, multifactor productivity growth over the 1987-2010 period has averaged 1.1 percent per year according to the Bureau of Labor Statistics (2011a).

---

[3]The sensitivity of these estimates can be determined by extrapolating the experience curve through labor force projections to age 90. The impact is around −0.008 percentage point using specifications for college graduates. Another adjustment would be to take into account unemployment rates by age, but the committee did not undertake this estimate.

TABLE 6-1 Projected Impact of Changing Age Distribution on Productivity for Two Education Groups, 2010-2020 and 2020-2030

Education Group	Impact of Changing Age Distribution on Productivity (percentage points per year)	
	2010-2020	2020-2030
High school		
Quartic fit	0.020	0.005
Actual	0.023	0.004
Quadratic specification	−0.013	0.006
College		
Quartic fit	0.006	0.011
Actual	−0.003	0.009
Quadratic specification	−0.010	0.024

Research indicates that changes in the age distribution of workers may impact relative wages. Card and Lemieux (2001) estimate that a 1 percent increase in the share of workers in a cohort relative to other workers will lower their earnings by approximately 0.2 percent for a given education and cohort, while Carneiro and Lee (2011) estimate an impact that is approximately one-half of that. The committee examined the impact of allowing imperfect substitutability on the age-productivity relationship. Dividing the workforce into six subgroups, it estimates that assuming perfect substitution among different age groups raises calculated productivity growth by 0.01 to 0.02 percentage points per year over the 2010-2030 period, depending upon which of the two estimates is used. In the context of all the factors at work, the substitution impact is very small.

The committee concludes that, taking earnings as a proxy for productivity, the impact of the changing age distribution on the level of productivity is negligible. The intuition behind these results can be explained using the quadratic specification of the earnings function for college graduates. According to the committee's projections, the average age of the labor force in the age range examined here is expected to increase by 2.0 years from 2010 to 2030. It estimates the slope of the log experience curve at the average experience for this period for college graduates is 1.2 percent per year of experience. Over the 20-year period, this averages $1.2 \times (2.0)/20 = 0.12$ percentage points per year. The estimates in Table 6-1 are slightly lower than this estimate because of asymmetries in the age distribution, but from an economic point of view the estimates are virtually identical. The impact of the changing age distribution on productivity is small fundamentally because the slope of the earnings curve at the current average age of the labor force is close to zero. In other words, if the average age of the workforce were to increase by a single year (and ignoring for simplicity the dispersion of worker ages), the impact of estimated productivity would be essentially nil.

Productivity and the Changing Distribution of the Workforce

In contrast to the vast enterprise engaged in estimating earnings-experience functions, there is very little research on the question of the impact of changes in the age distribution on overall productivity. An early study by Cutler et al. (1990) looked at the impact of changes in the growth rate of the labor force on labor productivity using a panel of countries over the period 1960-1985 and subperiods. After conducting a battery of tests, they conclude, "Because the annual labor force growth rate is predicted to fall by about 1 percentage point between 1990 and 2050, with most of the change occurring between 1990 and 2010, our estimates imply an increase of about 0.6 percentage point in annual productivity growth" (p. 43). When they correct for the average age of the labor force (similar to below), they find a slightly smaller impact. Their net results are that slower labor force growth accompanied by a higher average age leads to higher labor productivity.

More recent work by Feyrer (2007 and 2008) uses more detailed demographic data. His approach takes measures of productivity growth in major countries and combines them with estimates of the shares of the labor force in different age groups, using output data from the Penn World Table 6.0 and worker data from the International Labor Organization for decadal observations, the latter interpolated for 5-year intervals using population data from the United Nations. The total sample is 87 countries, while a more appropriate sample of countries for our purpose is limited to 21 OECD countries.

The Feyrer work shows an implausible pattern of coefficients when all six age groups are included. The ordinary least squares estimates for the OECD countries indicate that there is a logarithmic productivity bonus for workers in the 40-49 age group of 2.3 (a factor of 10) relative to workers aged 30-39 and of 2.0 (a factor of 8) relative to workers 50-59. These estimates likely reflect sampling error that arises from an excessive number of estimated parameters (i.e., equations that include all share variables). The committee therefore reestimated the productivity equations using linear, quadratic, and cubic functions of the average age.[4] This reestimation

---

[4]This analysis examines OECD countries only (total observations $N = 126$) because the other countries not only have poorer quality data but also seem less relevant to understanding productivity patterns in an aging society. If the equations for all countries are used, the estimated impact on productivity growth is a larger positive number than that shown in Table 6-2.

produced reasonable estimates, with a hump-shaped function of age that reaches a maximum at approximately 40 years.

For the sample of OECD countries, the United States lies pretty much in the mean of the sample of average ages. For the latest year (2000), the mean age of the U.S. workforce in the Feyrer data set is 40.1, while the range for OECD countries is 37.7 to 45.0 years. The average age of the workforce is estimated to increase from 41.1 years in 2010 to 43.2 years in 2030, so the mean value is within the range of estimates in the data used to estimate the productivity function.

Table 6-2 shows calculations analogous to those shown in Table 6-1 for the aggregate productivity equations. These equations estimate the impact of polynomial functions of the change in mean age on the change in the logarithm of total factor productivity using the Feyrer data set. For all three specifications, the committee has taken the mean age of the labor force from its estimated and projected age distributions for the years 2010, 2020, and 2030. If the equations are nested, the cubic term is statistically insignificant when the linear and quadratic terms are included (p = 0.46). The quadratic term is statistically significant when the linear term is included (p = 0.034). On a statistical basis, therefore, the committee prefers the quadratic specification in Table 6-2.

In the preferred equation, the change in the age distribution subtracts approximately 0.1 percent per year from aggregate productivity over the next two decades. However, this finding is sensitive to alternative specifications.

Conclusion on Productivity

The impact of changes in the composition of the labor force on productivity shows consistent results in all the committee's tests. Even though the numbers vary slightly depending on the technique, estimation period, and group, the estimates all indicate that the age composition effect on

TABLE 6-2 Projected Impact of Changing Age Distribution on Productivity Using Three Aggregate Productivity Estimates, 2010-2020 and 2020-2030

Productivity Estimates	Impact of Changing Age Distribution on Productivity (% change per year)	
	2010-2020	2020-2030
Linear	0.60	0.25
Quadratic	−0.06	−0.14
Cubic	0.09	0.04

productivity for the U.S. labor force over the next two decades is very small. The only exception is the linear productivity equation in Table 6-2, but this estimate should be discounted both because it is inconsistent with the earnings approach and because the quadratic approach has superior statistical qualities.

Therefore, the bottom line is that the committee's estimates indicate that there is likely to be a negligible effect of the age composition of the labor force on aggregate productivity over the next two decades. The summary judgment is that the age composition effect is between –0.1 and +0.1 percentage point per year.

However, these estimates are subject to some remaining uncertainty. For the earnings estimates, the uncertainties arise because of the concern that earnings do not reflect marginal productivities. If that relationship were clearly established, then the estimates in Table 6-1 indicate that the impact of the changing age distribution is close to zero. From a conceptual point of view, the productivity approach is superior because it would capture the substitution and complementarities among different groups as well as any externalities (at least in the sample period). However, at present, the empirical results are quite fragile and subject to specification concerns, so the results shown in Table 6-2 must be taken as very tentative.

IMPLICATIONS

The committee has considered the implications of its review of the relationship between the aging of the workforce and productivity and innovation. There are multiple pathways from a changing age distribution to the growth of productivity and income and their eventual magnitude. The most important in the long run is the rate of total factor productivity. The United States has been a major contributor to technological change, so it is important to ensure that policies are well-designed for innovation in an aging society.

One of the major policy levers on productivity and innovation is immigration. This is particularly important for scientists and innovators, where the United States has proven to be fertile soil for nurturing inventive talent, as was seen in the preceding discussion of the greatest scientists. Immigration has been a major source of scientific and innovative gains in this country over the last century. Immigration, and particularly the skill characteristics of immigration, is perhaps the most important way to affect innovativeness. Immigration policies must therefore be very sensitive to the potential for retarding the flow of the best talent to the United States.

Another factor that can play a particularly important role is the pattern of support for young scientists and engineers. This is an area where small changes in public policy and funding might have a large effect on creative outputs. While there has been attention paid to the lengthening time to the doctorate and the increased age at which scientists win their first grants, it appears that this is a particularly critical question for creative life spans. Earlier NRC studies discussed issues in this area, and the present committee would note two measures that are particularly important. First, it is important to ensure that young researchers have access to federal grants. This will be especially critical in an environment in which the federal budget is constrained and federal funds for science and engineering are likely to be under severe pressure. Additionally, it is important to ensure that the time to degree for young researchers be kept at the minimum so that they can progress to productive and independent scientific careers. This emphasizes the need for strong support for doctoral and postdoctoral scientists and engineers as well as measures that shorten the time during which young people are dependent on older researchers for support.

An important area for innovational structure is retirement policy. Fiscal concerns suggest that the country should support measures that encourage people to work longer. This is particularly true of incentives to retire early that have been discussed in Chapter 5 and elsewhere in this report. However, the committee would issue cautions about the potential squeeze on young scientists in a period in which universities and other institutions of innovation are under pressure. There has been aging in our innovational institutions over recent years, and this is of concern for a sector where the most innovative work is done early in the life cycle, as seen above. Attention to the needs of young scientists will help advance the early stages of scientific careers. Innovational institutions should pay increased attention to the need to ensure that there is ample room for young scientists and scholars in their ranks.

Finally, some federal spending and tax structures are more likely to promote innovation than others. Programs to support education, science programs, and scholarships for college and postgraduate students are better at creating an innovative society than many existing federal programs. It is important that fiscal decisions in a constrained budget environment be mindful of the impact of policies on innovation and adaptiveness.

7

Saving and Retirement Security

This chapter addresses two broad questions related to saving and retirement security in the United States in the face of population aging: (1) How is population aging likely to affect national saving rates, levels of retirement wealth and income, and retirement security? and (2) What are some policy options for mitigating potential negative effects that population aging may have on retirement security?

Saving is a key factor shaping the economic well-being of individuals and the nation as a whole. Households need saving for many reasons, including precautionary ones (to guard against large, unexpected costs or job loss), to accumulate assets for major purchases, and to prepare for retirement. At the macroeconomic level, national saving contributes to the amount of capital available for production and hence for economic growth.

As our society ages, household saving and dissaving (spending) patterns can be expected to change in a number of ways, with a variety of consequences for national saving. For instance, as people age and move into retirement, many will begin liquidating their stock of retirement assets to generate income that pays for living expenses, health care, and retirement care, among other things. Accordingly, as the percentage of the population in retirement grows relative to the rest of the population, the cumulative effect of such disinvestment may place downward pressure on the value of equities, housing, and other assets held by the older population. If older members of the population have different risk preferences and favor different asset classes than younger people—for instance, if they are more averse to risk—then an aging population can produce a shift in aggregate taste for risk and a new sharing of risk between cohorts. Additional pressure on retirement income security may come from policy changes that address the excess of current government promises to pay Social Security, Medicare, and Medicaid over the projected tax revenues available to fund those programs.

In the absence of public policy reforms or new government programs, some households will be able to take steps to mitigate the negative effects that population aging may have on their retirement security. People may elect to work longer, save more, reallocate assets to less risky investments, change retirement consumption plans, or diversify retirement-related risks through the purchase of annuities or other insurance products—for example, long-term care insurance. Yet governments, too, can promote retirement security by adopting a holistic view of retirement policy that ensures that negative impacts from prospective reform of support systems are at least partially offset by policies and programs that strengthen household saving and the workplace-based retirement system.

The committee begins by reviewing data on U.S. saving and wealth patterns and showing that current private and public saving rates by and for workers are probably inadequate to provide a level of future retirement resources similar to that of recent retirees. While such a resource shortfall will result in economic stress on households, governments, and the macroeconomy, these concerns are not insurmountable. Nevertheless, addressing them effectively will require a renewed partnership between households, employers, and the government to ensure that retirement risk burdens are distributed fairly and that future generations of workers have a secure retirement.

DEFINING RETIREMENT WEALTH AND SAVING

To provide context for the rest of the chapter, the committee begins by examining how national and household wealth in the United States, as well as saving rates and retirement adequacy, have changed over the recent past. As will be seen, personal household saving has increased of late, but these patterns are offset by the largest federal budget deficits in decades.

Measuring Household and National Wealth

Gross national wealth (or worth) equals the total value of national assets (financial and nonfinancial) in an economy. Net national wealth, as defined in the Federal Reserve's *Flow of Funds Accounts* (2011), is equal to total assets less total liabilities; this metric provides a broad-based measure of resources available to finance future consumption. Figure 7-1 shows the evolution of real (2005 dollars) net worth for the period 1960-2010, and indicates that Americans' real net worth grew steadily over the past

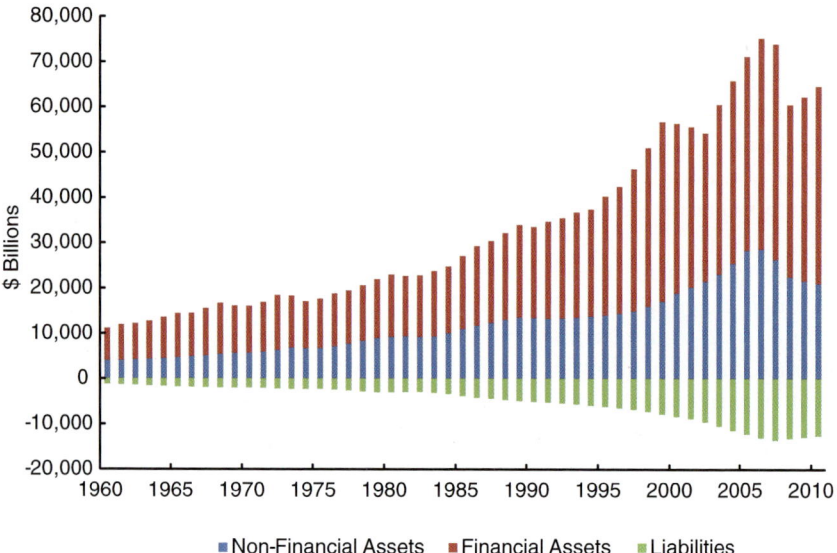

FIGURE 7-1 Components of household real net worth, 1960-2010 (in 2005 dollars). SOURCE: Federal Reserve (2011).

50 years, averaging 3.5 percent annually and experiencing only 11 years of decline. Figure 7-1 suggests that growth in net wealth is correlated with the real business cycle.

National Saving Patterns

To effectively discuss saving and the impact of an aging society on saving, the committee distinguishes between private and government saving. The portion of a nation's income not used for consumption is the sum of both kinds of saving, and it is termed national saving. In the United States, national saving and its component parts are typically measured using data from the National Income and Product Accounts (NIPA) drawn from the Bureau of Economic Analysis (BEA) (2011). Figure 7-2 shows the relationship between U.S. net private and public saving and net national saving over the past half-century. The evidence indicates that net national saving as a percent of U.S. gross domestic product (GDP) has declined in the last half-century, and this decline is attributable to declines in both private and government saving. A discussion of different saving concepts is provided in the attachment to this chapter.

The BEA defines private saving as the sum of business and personal saving, where "personal" includes not just households but also nonprofit

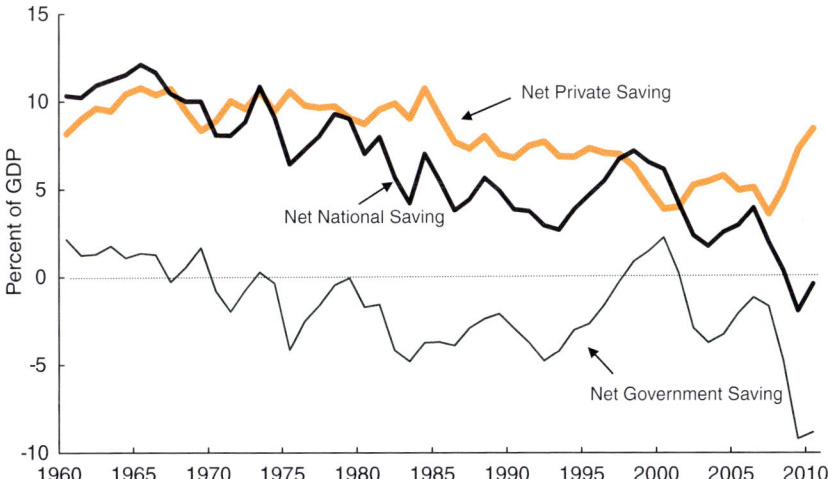

FIGURE 7-2 Net national saving, 1960-2010. SOURCE: Bureau of Economic Analysis.

entities such as foundations, churches, and charities. Personal saving is defined as the difference between personal income and the sum of personal outlays and personal current taxes. Accordingly, the personal saving rate divides the flow of dollars saved by disposable personal income; this is the standard measure of personal saving in the United States (Guidolin and La Jeunesse, 2007). Over the last 50 years, there were three distinct periods, as depicted in Figure 7-3. The 1960-1985 period was characterized by relatively high personal saving rates, the 1985-2005 period was characterized by rapidly declining personal saving rates, and the last 5 years (2006-2011) have seen steadily increasing personal saving rates. Over the 25-year period 1961-1985, personal saving rates averaged 9.2 percent; they were never lower than 7.8 percent (1969) and peaked in 1982 for a post-Second World War high of 10.9 percent. By contrast, in the subsequent 25-year span, the average personal saving rate was only about 4.8 percent, declining in 19 of 25 years and sinking to a 70-year low of 1.5 percent in 2005.

The other main form of saving is public or government saving, measured as the difference between government revenues and expenditures. If public expenditures exceed government revenues, the public sector must borrow funds to make up the difference, which in turn may decrease funds available for private investment. At the federal level, there are few constraints on the amount of borrowing that is permitted. In contrast to the federal government, most state governments use capital budgeting rules for capital expenditures, and many have balanced budget requirements for their

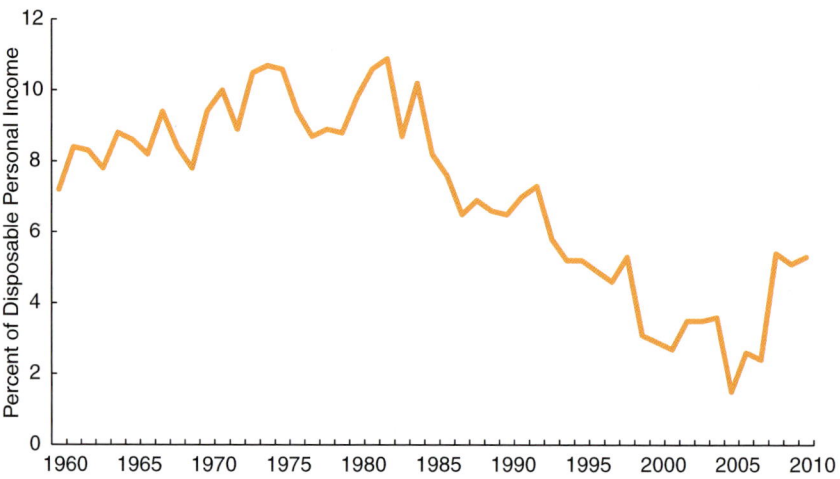

FIGURE 7-3 Personal saving rate, 1960-2010. SOURCE: Bureau of Economic Analysis.

current operating budgets.[1] Overall, state and local government contributions to national saving (or dissaving) tend to be relatively small relative to GDP. Figure 7-4 shows net government saving over the 1960-2010 period and demonstrates that total net government saving is strongly correlated with net federal saving. Indeed, state and local government saving rates have averaged about 0.38 percent of GDP over the past 50 years, ranging from a high of 1.25 percent in 1972 to a low of negative 0.55 percent in 2009. These figures, however, do not take into account the implicit borrowing associated with the underfunding in public pension plans (Novy-Marx and Rauh, 2010) or the underfunding of retiree health care promises. Accordingly, the states cannot be said to have contributed to net saving over the last quarter century when their off-balance-sheet shortfalls are taken into account.

The federal government has experienced rather wide swings in expenditures versus revenues over time: It ran small budget surpluses through much of the 1960s, posted small deficits through most of the 1970s, and then ran increasingly larger deficits through the 1980s and into the early 1990s. Between 1998 and 2001, the federal government ran small surpluses; it then began incurring deficits again in 2002. So while the average federal deficit was about 2.1 percent of GDP over the past half-century, federal govern-

---

[1] State balanced budget restrictions can be misleading because off-budget accounts such as defined benefit pensions and retiree health care benefits are often underfunded.

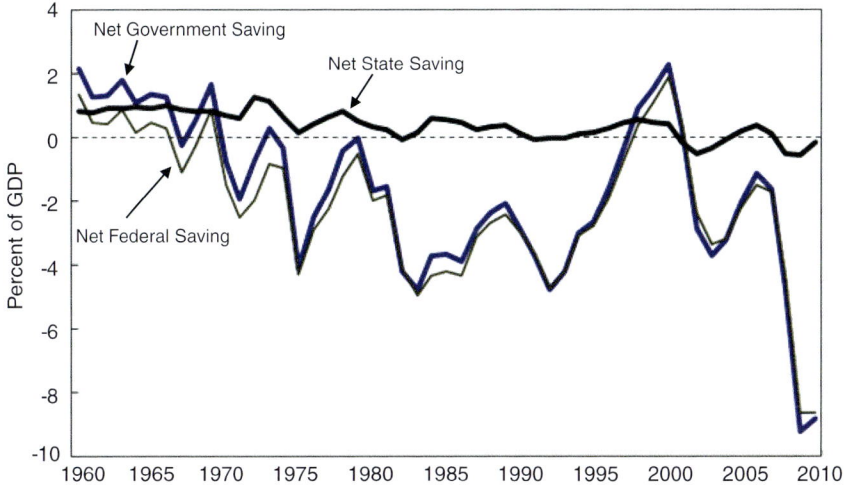

FIGURE 7-4 Net government saving, 1960-2010. SOURCE: Bureau of Economic Analysis.

ment net saving has ranged from a low of around negative 8.7 percent in 2010 to a high of about 1.9 percent in 2000. The historically large deficits of the last 3 years, in part caused by efforts to help the economy recover from the deep recession that followed the financial crisis in 2008, have unfortunately coincided with the leading edge of the retirement of the baby boom generation.

Looking ahead, these and other obligations will exert pressure on budgets at both the federal and state and local levels. Moreover, these figures do not include the enormous and persistent increases in the unfunded obligations scheduled under the Social Security and Medicare programs.[2] Some researchers have estimated that total underfunding of both Social Security and Medicare under current law stands at a present value of $9.5 trillion (over a 75-year horizon); the committee recognizes, however, that there is considerable controversy about these numbers and uncertainty associated

---

[2]The term "unfunded obligations" (or "unfunded liabilities") is used here as a means of describing the shortfall of projected revenues compared to scheduled benefit payments. The committee recognizes that, by law, there is no unfunded liability for either Social Security or Medicare Hospital Insurance: Actual law prohibits spending anything on these two programs in excess of accumulated reserves and current revenues. The reason that economists and finance experts regularly measure the shortfall or "implicit" debt of these programs is because this is a sensible way to evaluate the potential burden of "keeping the promises." To ignore the shortfall between scheduled and payable benefits would be highly misleading.

with such estimates.[3] Nevertheless, under current law, benefit projections will contribute to large and rising future federal obligations.

National Saving and an Aging Society

The recent financial crisis and recession have taken a severe toll on household wealth and national saving. Total net national saving has dropped substantially, owing to the historically large federal deficits and the accompanying large decrease in public saving. The stock of household wealth has also declined owing to the sharp decline in home prices, along with the need for millions of Americans to tap into their retirement saving owing to high unemployment.

Taking a longer-term perspective, it is difficult to predict the likely impact of population aging on national patterns of wealth accumulation. The simple economic life-cycle model predicts that people save during their working lives and draw down this wealth during retirement. For this reason, some suggest that baby boomer retirees will need to sell off their assets so as to finance consumption, which might prompt a market meltdown. On the other hand, because population aging is predictable, economic theory suggests current asset prices will adjust so that expected returns will be positive over all future time periods. Furthermore, the demand for assets by emerging economies (some of which are experiencing slower or no population aging) may help offset the sales of assets by economies with older populations (for more on such possibilities, see Chapter 8). It is also uncertain how the savings of the young and middle-aged will respond to changes brought on by an aging population. They may save at a higher rate than past generations if they anticipate reductions in public health and retirement benefits and increased longevity. On the other hand, they might save less if they plan on working longer, thus needing a relatively smaller nest egg in retirement.

It is also worth pointing out that the mix and type of saving instru-

---

[3]The $9.5 trillion is a so-called "open-group" measure, which takes into account system Trust Funds as well as scheduled future taxes and benefits. By contrast, a closed-group measure of unfunded liabilities includes projected benefits and taxes only for persons aged 15+ (in other words, those under age 15 or as yet unborn are excluded). According to this second measure, the closed-group Social Security unfunded value comes to $18.8 trillion, including the combined Trust Funds; excluding them, the unfunded amount would be $21.3 trillion (Board of Trustees, Federal Old-Age and Survivors Insurance and Federal Disability Insurance Trust Funds, 2011, p. 67). Medicare closed-group as well as open-group values are more uncertain since the system has a call on general revenues and because uncertainties about the impact of the health care reform bill make cost-savings difficult to compute (Boards of Trustees, Federal Hospital Insurance and Federal Supplementary Medical Insurance Trust Funds, 2011).

ments demanded by an aging population are likely to differ from those desired in the past (Mitchell et al., 2006). For instance, the long-term movement toward defined contribution (DC) pensions and away from defined benefit (DB) pension plans is likely to focus older individuals on new ways to manage their spending patterns and draw down their wealth throughout retirement. Guaranteed annuities represent an appealing mechanism by which older persons can protect themselves against outliving their assets, and future demand is likely to increase for products that can help make retirement income more predictable (Chai et al., 2011). Each of these is likely to challenge financial firms to design new products to provide the desired balance between protection from risk and higher expected returns. Another set of risks against which financial protection may be desired is political risk: the huge underfunded liabilities of public pension and many retiree health care plans in the United States leave those programs susceptible to reductions in scheduled benefits or other changes to reduce costs. That uncertainty may induce the young and old alike to take precautionary steps, such as by planning to work longer, saving more, and drawing down assets less quickly than they would have otherwise. While there is little hard evidence on this, early results suggest that such patterns are already evident in the wake of the financial crisis (Coronado and Dynan, in press).

An important dimension to the impact of aging on national saving is the fact that households differ greatly in terms of their standards of living. Households with low levels of human capital and low lifetime earnings will almost certainly continue to save little and to rely heavily on social programs to maintain their standard of living. It is also likely that households with higher lifetime earnings will need to be prepared to maintain an increasing share of their retirement living standards through their own means rather than through government programs. Research suggests that this may already be occurring, with households in the top quartile of earnings relying less on government social welfare programs for retirement income than previous generations of households in this quartile (Purcell, 2009a). One challenge of an aging population may be a growing number of increasingly long-lived individuals who outlive their retirement resources and will then rely heavily on the social safety net to meet late-life needs (see Table 7-1).

ARE SAVING RATES SUFFICIENT IN VIEW OF POPULATION AGING?

This section asks whether household saving rates are adequate in view of population aging, and it identifies which subsets of people are at risk of falling behind.

TABLE 7-1 Distribution of Household Wealth from Pensions, Social Security, and Other Sources, by Wealth Decile: Early Boomers Aged 51-56 in 2004 (in 2010 dollars)

Source	Wealth Decile Poorest 1	2	3	4	5	6	7	8	9	Wealthiest 10	Average
Pension wealth	2,445	11,531	33,412	59,120	108,255	139,015	206,486	280,263	402,127	595,128	178,007
Social Security wealth	65,819	125,364	163,678	213,629	211,623	237,545	248,236	261,890	285,379	289,698	208,096
Other wealth	6,730	36,034	81,427	114,054	180,050	266,219	345,428	481,462	700,225	1,544,980	360,822
Total wealth	74,994	172,929	278,517	386,802	499,927	642,779	800,150	1,023,615	1,387,731	2,429,807	746,924
Pension wealth/total wealth (%)	3	7	12	15	22	22	26	27	29	24	24
Social Security wealth/total wealth (%)	88	72	59	55	42	37	31	26	21	12	28

NOTE: Households with the top and bottom 1 percent of total wealth are excluded.
SOURCE: Derived by Olivia S. Mitchell and Yong Yu from data from the Health and Retirement Study provided in Gustman, Steinmeier, and Tabatai (2010).

Defining Adequacy

The adequacy of retirement security is usually judged using two different measures. The first focuses on a retiree's income flow compared to his preretirement income flow and asks whether retirees' living standards are close to what they experienced during their working life. The second measure focuses on the sufficiency of retirement resources, or the stock of assets available to smooth lifetime well-being. In either case, one must assess saving patterns, returns earned on invested assets, the number of years spent accumulating retirement assets, the period expected in retirement, and the mix of anticipated retirement income and assets. In the absence of Social Security, these two dimensions of adequacy are highly correlated because having sufficient retirement resources is crucial to generating adequate retirement income to support retirement consumption. Yet the progressivity of the current Social Security benefit structure means that some households with low lifetime earnings will require fewer of their own retirement assets to achieve adequacy. Figure 7-5 compares sources of income for the top and bottom quartile of Americans over the age of 64 for the years 1975 and 2008. The findings suggest that the bottom quartile continues to rely heavily on Social Security benefits (about 84 percent of income in 2008), whereas the top quartile has grown less reliant on Social Security payments

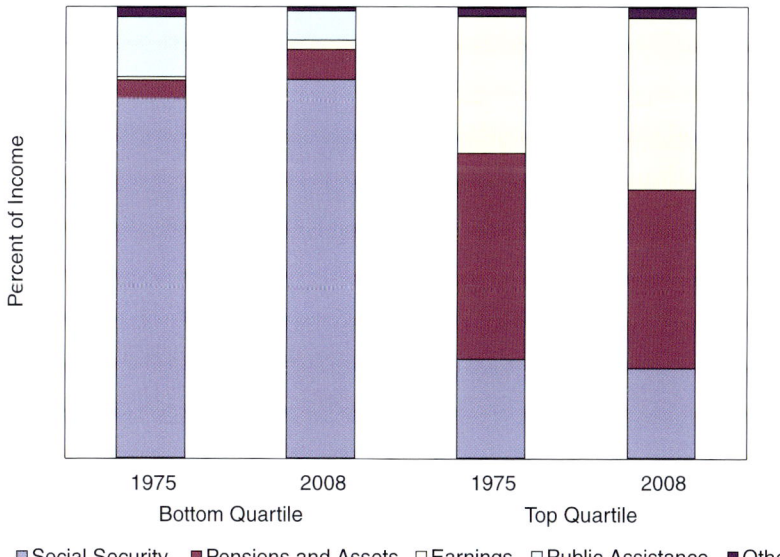

FIGURE 7-5 Income distribution, by source, for people aged 65+ in the top and bottom income quartiles, 1975 and 2008. SOURCE: Purcell (2009a).

(about 20 percent of income in 2008). Yet by 2008, the bottom quartile had become relatively more reliant on its own assets as a source of income, and both groups experienced an increase in reliance on labor earnings over time.

Empirical Approaches and Aggregate Findings

Analysts disagree about whether and which Americans are adequately prepared for retirement in terms of resources and retirement income. To explain this conundrum, it is important to point out that economists and financial advisers measure adequacy in different ways. One methodology uses a target saving measure to determine adequacy. This methodology defines projected retirement expenditure levels for a given household and specifies the mix of income and assets required to cover a proportion (or all) of this target spending level. Accordingly, if a household seems likely to accumulate enough assets to support this level of consumption, the household's plan is said to be adequate; otherwise it will have a shortfall and additional saving needed may be specified to hit the target. Authors who use this approach generally conclude that a majority of Americans will face shortfalls in retirement, due to insufficient saving and early retirement (Schieber, 2004; Mitchell and Moore, 1998; McGill et al., 2010). In other words, they have not accumulated assets sufficiently rapidly to achieve the replacement rate goal. Mitchell and Moore (1998) conclude that most older households have accumulated far too little to replace preretirement income if they plan on retiring at age 62; in fact they would need to save on average 18 percent more per year (above current saving rates) to attain the desired asset level. Deferring retirement to age 65 would cut the shortfall in half.

A variant on this approach focuses on whether retirees have command over resources sufficient to replace 70-75 percent of preretirement (post-tax) income. Of course this presumes that peoples' actual preretirement consumption levels are adequate, and that having a drop in spending of one-quarter in retirement would not cause hardship. For example, Munnell and Soto (2005) use the Health and Retirement Study (HRS) to estimate how much income households receive in retirement relative to earnings before retirement. They take into account all actual and potential sources of income, including pensions, Social Security, and home equity, and conclude that replacement rates for households with employment-based pensions are 79 percent for couples and 89 percent for single-person households. Replacement rates for households without pensions are 62 percent and 63 percent, respectively.

A second approach to the adequacy question uses economic optimization models to evaluate whether people have accumulated enough to smooth their lifetime well-being. A widely cited analysis by Scholz, Seshadri, and Khitatrakun (2006) develops a life-cycle model to calculate optimal saving decisions for HRS households, taking into account longevity risk, income shocks, medical expenses, taxes and transfers, pension and social security benefits, and changes in family composition. After deriving estimates of wealth that the households would ideally amass, they compare these outcomes with observed wealth patterns. Since peoples' ideal wealth accumulation patterns are highly correlated with actual wealth patterns, the authors conclude that most people were doing approximately the "right thing." While some 20 percent did appear to have saved too little, the amount of undersaving was generally small. In contrast, using a similar model but an earlier data set, Bernheim (1997) found that baby boomers had accumulated only about one-third as much financial and housing wealth as they should have.

In sum, depending on the specific study, research suggests that between one-fifth and two-thirds of the older population can be said to have undersaved for retirement. Moreover, these studies assume that Social Security and Medicare benefits will be paid as scheduled.[4] Since this is improbable (see Chapter 9), the chances of shortfalls are likely even greater.

Disaggregating Adequacy Measures

Conclusions about savings adequacy might be more similar if such differences could be reconciled (Haveman et al., 2007). But in any event, all analysts agree that there is much heterogeneity in retirement wealth and consequently adequacy. One factor differentiating those who save from those who do not is financial literacy; as Lusardi and Mitchell (2011) show, the least financially literate are also least likely to plan for retirement and to actually execute successful saving plans. As noted in the preceding section, however, accumulating few liquid financial assets may be rational for low-income individuals to the extent that they expect to receive relatively generous benefits from Social Security along with means-tested (e.g., Medicaid) benefits. In other words, it may be economically sensible for the low-income population to save little even if it leaves it exposed to financial shocks.

---

[4]Mitchell and Moore (1997) found that the median HRS black and Hispanic households on the verge of retirement in 1992 had only $5,000 in financial wealth; by contrast whites had approximately 11 times more financial wealth, and more than four times as much wealth when housing is included. For all racial groupings, at the median, housing wealth comprised over half of wealth. Its importance was greatest for black and Hispanic households, where housing equity represented the vast majority of accessible wealth. Using 2001 data, Wolfe (2006) concluded that for those aged 47-64, whites had 5.5 times the net worth of nonwhites. Somewhat offsetting the lower wealth levels for nonwhites is their lower survival rates: After controlling for both race and education, Wolfe predicted that the odds of death for black men were 1.3 times those for other groups. Nevertheless, for those aged 65-90, black men were not found to have a significantly higher risk of death than other males. For additional views see Waldron (2002).

Another factor is that low-income households may be at greater risk because a larger proportion of their retirement income is used to replace necessities. One study found that replacement rates need to be as high as 94 percent for households earning $20,000 or less per year, while those earning $60,000-$90,000 have replacement rates of about 78 percent to achieve retirement adequacy (Aon Consulting, 2008). It also appears that employees with defined contribution plans were once less likely to save over their lifetimes, though those covered by defined benefit pensions can also fall short due to insufficient pension funding (McGill et al., 2010). Workers in the not-for-profit sector do appear to be saving enough to accumulate adequate retirement assets (Hammond and Richardson, 2009), particularly the longer-tenured employees.

The fact that the cost of medical care continues to outpace both earnings and overall price increases indicates that this component of retirement spending will remain substantially uncertain into the future. Many current projections indicate that retirees will need to devote an increasing fraction of retirement resources to paying for health care, as the Medicare and Medicaid systems along with employer-provided retiree health insurance face solvency pressures. If reforms in these systems result in less generous public health insurance benefits, this could reverse the long-term trend of retirees bearing a declining share of responsibility for their health-related expenses (Richardson, 2008). Even prior to the reforms, the Employee Benefit Research Institute (2009) projected that workers retiring in 2009 would need as much as $378,000 (for males; $450,000 for females) to be 90 percent sure of having enough assets to pay for out-of-pocket health care costs in retirement. If accurate, these estimates suggest many current workers are quite likely to be undersaving for a secure old age.

Handling Risk During Retirement

Whether workers and retirees have adequate retirement provision depends in large part on the risks people will face, which in turn suggests that understanding retirement risks is critical to predicting whether retirement accumulations will be adequate. Many older households are increasingly being asked to decide how much to save, where to invest, when to claim benefits, and how to effectively protect against longevity risk and potentially large macroeconomic shocks. Public policy and the markets have made some progress in helping people to better manage these risks by rolling out pension autoenrollment, autoescalation, and life-cycle default funds. Yet the typical U.S. pension contribution threshold is still too low to ensure adequate retirement wealth, and life-cycle funds can be susceptible to market volatility and systemic shocks.

Investment Portfolio Risk

One question that has interested researchers for decades is whether and how people's risk tolerance, and hence investment and insurance demand, changes with age. Interestingly, theory and evidence are still inconclusive regarding this question; some analysts predict that equity holding will fall with age, while others find the opposite. On the whole, there is little agreement in the literature about whether an aging population will liquidate equity holdings en masse. In practice there are many different assets available to investors, with different risk attributes and correspondingly different expected returns. In general, investors require a higher rate of return on assets that have more market or aggregate risk, which is risk that cannot be avoided through portfolio diversification. For example, the expected rate of return on a diversified portfolio of stocks is higher than that on a portfolio of Treasury securities, because investors are averse to the risk that the stocks will perform poorly just when the rest of the economy is also weak. The difference between the expected return on risky stocks and Treasury bills is called the "equity risk premium." Other risky investments, such as corporate bonds and real estate, also have expected returns in excess of Treasury rates because they expose investors to undiversifiable risks.

As the population ages, it is possible that such demographic change will affect the aggregate risk appetite of the capital market. If an older population is more risk averse than a younger one, the price of risky assets could be lower and required risk premiums commensurately higher than in the past. An increase in demand for relatively safe financial assets would create incentives for companies to shift to investing in safer real projects as well, causing shifts in the production process and in the mix of goods and services produced. An increase in risk aversion at older ages could be induced by changing economic circumstances, or it could arise from fundamental changes in preferences. Several studies, notably Bodie, Merton, and Samuelson (1992) and Jagannathan and Kocherlakota (1996), have suggested that older households should be less tolerant of investment risk because they cannot offset adverse shocks to the value of their asset holdings by increasing their labor supply. The typical advice of financial advisers to reduce exposure to investment risk with age is consistent with that reasoning. Yet more recent analyses have suggested that the link between age and the tolerance for investment risk—and its relation to labor income—may be more complicated. Benzoni, Collin-Dufresne, and Goldstein (2007) argue that because labor income is a significant source of long-run market risk for young people, they are expected to be more averse to investment risk than middle-aged households, whose lifetime labor income is less uncertain. This study predicts a hump-shaped pattern of risky asset holding over the life cycle, which in aggregate would imply greater risk tolerance when a larger portion of the population is middle-aged. A life-cycle perspective that includes housing, such as that developed by Bakshi and Chen (1994), also suggests that the demand for financial assets may increase as people age and their demand for housing diminishes.[5] It is more difficult to evaluate whether aging causes fundamental changes in preferences toward risk, and there has been relatively little work done by economists on that question.[6]

Morbidity Risks

An aging society will also have an increasing likelihood of morbidity risks, as a growing percentage of the population is at an age where the incidence of multiple diseases, disorders, and medical conditions increases substantially (Chapter 4). Who will bear the risk burden for financing a population with this growing number of morbidities? Some have argued for a universal-coverage national health care insurance program with mandatory participation that would result in young healthy people bearing a larger share of risk burden of paying for older people's health care costs. Even under present law, as people age, they tend to become more dependent on government health care programs, so an aging population will likely generate increasing pressure on the Medicare and Medicaid systems, leading to the potential of ever-increasing shifts of elderly health-related risk burdens onto the working age population in an attempt to maintain system solvency. And to the extent that Social Security and Medicare provide a floor of protection to the elderly, financial market shocks that impact older people's ability to pay for their own needs will also likely shift an increasing share of these burdens onto the labor force. Financing the costs of this shift in elderly health-related risk burdens can be facilitated through new taxes on and transfers from the labor force, but *ex ante* it is virtually impossible to quantify what these political risks will be and how they will be allocated.

---

[5]It is also important to recognize that risk tolerance is not spread evenly among individuals or households within age groups. Much of the total wealth of older people is held by those with very high wealth. However, the pattern of risk tolerance among the very wealthy is not clear from previous research. Older studies (e.g., Riley and Chow, 1992; Morin and Suarez, 1983) conclude that risk aversion declines with age. More recent studies (Wang and Hanna, 1997; Paravisini, Rappoport, and Ravine, 2010) find that wealthier investors are more risk averse. And, any number of studies (e.g., Hariharana, Chapman, and Domian, 2000; Hanna and Lindamood, 2004; Lybbert and Just, 2007; Kapteyn and Teppa, 2011) question the quality/usefulness of existing measures of risk tolerance and note problems associated with empirical tests of the relationship between wealth and risk aversion.

[6]There have been studies of the impact of changes in family status such as widowhood or divorce, where there is usually a large negative impact on income and assets. And there is separate research on the health/wealth trajectory with age. As far as the committee knows, there is no thorough and overarching analysis of how the riskiness of household assets changes with age for the elderly.

Social Security and Medicare Solvency Risk

When forecasting the contribution rate needed to achieve retirement security, most academic studies and financial planning simulation models assume that Social Security and Medicare scheduled benefits will continue to be paid. Yet this is by no means assured in view of the projected insolvency of these systems given current payroll tax and benefit formulas (Board of Trustees, Federal Old-Age and Survivors Insurance and Federal Disability Insurance Trust Funds, 2011). Payroll tax collections for Social Security benefits have been insufficient to cover annual cost from 2010; after Trust Fund assets are exhausted, payroll tax revenue will be sufficient to pay only about 75 percent of scheduled benefits beginning around 2036.

Older Americans' ability to rely on the Medicare system is also in doubt. Medicare's health insurance (HI) expenditures have exceeded HI Trust Fund income annually since 2008 and are projected to continue doing so until the HI Trust Fund is exhausted, in 2024. While household premium and general tax revenue income are reset each year to match expected costs, the projected cost growth of Medicare Parts B and D will require households and government to devote ever increasing shares of their budgets to financing these benefits.

Policy makers have not agreed on the feasible set of public policy solutions for restoring the solvency of these systems. Possible reforms include increasing payroll taxes by changing either the tax rate or tax base (or a combination of both), cutting the level or growth of benefits, raising the minimum age for normal and early benefit eligibility, expansion of means testing, or some combination of these. Because Social Security and Medicare currently provide a great deal of purchasing power for a substantial percentage of the population (SSA, 2010b), such profound uncertainty makes it difficult to judge future retiree adequacy with any confidence. The risk of inadequacy is substantial for the bottom quartile of workers, who rely most heavily on Social Security and Medicare, and threatens to reverse the decades-long trend of declining elderly poverty rates (see Box 7-1). Yet system reforms will likely impact the retirement security of all cohorts, and offsetting reforms to other programs such as the employment-based retirement system will be needed to ensure that older Americans can maintain a reasonable standard of living during retirement.

One might ask why poverty rates among the elderly are not higher if many people save inadequately for retirement. This report notes that retirement adequacy is usually measured either by (1) focusing on a retiree's income flow compared to pre-retirement income, and asking whether the retiree's living standard is close to that experienced during the working life, or (2) focusing on the sufficiency of retirement resources, or the stock of assets available to smooth lifetime wellbeing. This is different from most

> **BOX 7-1**
> **Poverty Among the Elderly**
>
> Inadequate retirement saving and poor risk management increase the likelihood that a person will spend at least a portion of retired life in poverty. Using the U.S. government's official poverty line, poverty rates among the elderly have declined long-term (Wentworth and Pattison, 2002). Another study focused on more recent changes (Issa and Zedlewski, 2011, p. 5):
>
>> The Great Recession, which began in December 2007, reduced incomes and increased poverty for younger Americans. Between 2007 and 2009, the poverty rate for those younger than 65 increased from 18.0 to 20.7 percent. For adults age 65 or older, however, poverty rates fell from 9.7 to 8.9 percent, and the share living in low-income families fell from 36.1 to 33.7 percent [see Figure 7-1-1]. Old-age poverty declined primarily because Social Security's cost-of-living adjustment formula increased benefits by 5.8 percent in January 2009 (following a temporary surge in prices in mid-2008), while the price level fell slightly in 2009. This benefit increase significantly boosted incomes for low-income older adults, who rely primarily on Social Security. Poverty and near-poverty rates for adults age 75 or older declined more than for adults younger than 75 because Social Security makes up a larger share of their incomes. The incidence of near poverty fell slightly between 2007 and 2009—0.2 percentage points—among adults age 65 to 74. Their poverty rate fell more sharply, from 8.8 to 8.1 percent.
>
> Still another study (Short, 2011) computed new poverty numbers using a broader definition of income, and it finds poverty among the 65+ group to be 15.9 percent, versus 15.6 percent for those aged 10-64. The new measure differs from the official poverty line as follows (p. 8): "The official poverty measure does not take account of

concepts/measurements of poverty. It is quite conceivable that many people could save too little yet not be in poverty. One of the goals of the follow-on study to this report will be to quantify inadequacy according to different definitions and measurements and thereby obtain a better understanding of the relationship between poverty and retirement saving.

Workplace Retirement Income Plan Risk

Americans' retirement saving adequacy is strongly influenced by whether people participate in a workplace retirement income program. In the United States, pensions are usually of the DB or DC variety, though a plan may also be structured as a hybrid with both DB and DC characteristics. Employers who sponsor a DB plan typically offer coverage to most employees and require participation in the plan.[7] Private sector employers

---

[7] It should be noted that while a DB plan generally offers broad coverage, workers may lose any rights to pension benefits if they leave the organization that sponsors the plan. In other words, there is individual risk in DB plans associated with worker mobility.

taxes or of in-kind benefits aimed at improving the economic situation of the poor." So the usual view that poverty is lower among the elderly than among the nonelderly is sensitive to the definitions used (e.g., the inclusion or exclusion of Medicare premiums).

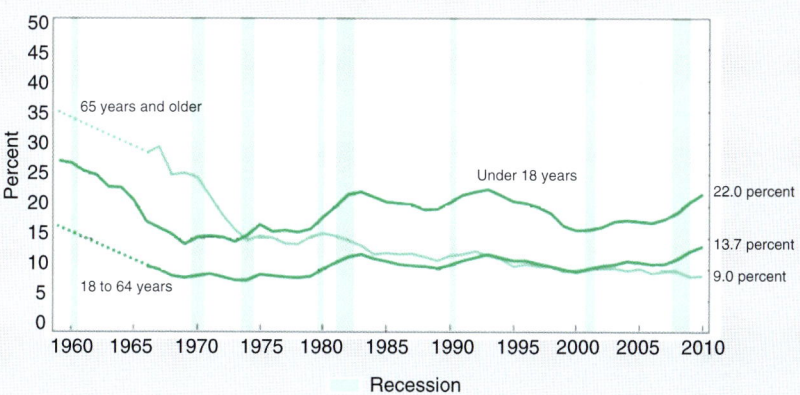

FIGURE 7-1-1 Poverty rates among three age groups, 1959-2010. SOURCE: U.S. Census Bureau, Current Population Survey 1960 to 2011, Annual Social and Economic Supplements.

are also responsible for maintaining minimum funding levels that reduce the risk that plan assets will fall short of promised payments. By contrast, DC plans typically have voluntary participation, and they allow employee elective contributions and choice over the investment of their retirement assets.

As discussed in Chapter 5, prior generations of American workers who had workplace coverage typically had a primary DB and may have had a supplemental DC plan. Beginning in the early 1980s, however, plan type became more sector-specific, with the majority of private-sector and federal government workers covered by a primary DC plan, while most state and local public sector workers continued to have a primary DB plan. Both types of plans are under considerable stress today. In DB plans, underfunding is widespread, partly because public pensions are generally not subject to federal minimum funding requirements. Moreover, though corporate DB plans have funding requirements, there is in fact widespread underfunding in this sector as well. In DC plans, low contribution rates (which result in inadequate retirement assets) are more prevalent in the for-profit sector's 401(k)-type DC plans than in the not-for-profit sector's DC-type plans.

Followers of workplace-based pensions have noted some positive, but also some negative, trends of late. In any year, about half the private sector workforce has been covered by employer pensions for three decades (Employee Benefit Research Institute, 2011a and 2011b), in spite of numerous legislative attempts to enhance coverage. Low-wage workers who change jobs often or work in small firms often lack the option to save in DC plans, giving rise to government proposals to expand coverage (Iwry, 2004). Nevertheless, several policy reforms have increased employer adoption of auto-enrollment and default provisions that boost DC plan participation and contributions. Employers who offer retirement plan contribution and investment defaults generally see higher pension saving rates (only partly offset by reductions in voluntary nonpension saving; Card and Ransom, 2011). As noted above, DB plans are suffering from the market downturn and persistent underfunding.[8] Regulatory burdens are widely believed to have restricted the growth and deepening of the employer-sponsored pension marketplace (Perun and Steuerle, 2006). In light of the budget stringencies discussed above, it would seem difficult to enhance tax inducements to boost pension saving. Nonetheless, if workplace retirement plans are to play a continued key role in helping the working-age population prepare for retirement, it will be critical for employers to adopt and support well-designed retirement plans that encourage workers to save adequately in diversified portfolios, which can maximize the likelihood of providing a secure retirement.

Housing Wealth Risk

In many nations, people have often considered housing as a safe asset, and U.S. baby boomers are no exception; they have relied more on housing equity for retirement security than previous generations (Lusardi and Mitchell, 2007a). Unfortunately, the bursting of the housing price bubble and ongoing housing market slump have eroded the large pool of retirement wealth that had been held in the form of home equity. Both the illiquidity of housing assets and the volatility of house prices can also affect the adequacy of retirement resources when retirees plan to lean heavily on housing wealth as a source of consumption. Real net household nonfinancial wealth experienced an approximately 26 percent decline since its peak in 2006. Such an extraordinary loss of wealth affects current and future retirees' ability

---

[8]DB plans are significantly subsidized currently by underpriced insurance premiums, and they are likely to face premium increases (as proposed in the President's 2012 budget), which may discourage employers from offering DB plans in the future. The government reinsurance entity, the Pension Benefit Guaranty Corporation, is itself rather seriously underfunded (see Pension Benefit Guaranty Corporation, 2011).

to rely on housing wealth to finance retirement consumption. In addition, many households enter retirement still holding a mortgage (Webb, 2009); this subjects them to additional pressure to generate adequate retirement assets to cover mortgage payments, and it also increases the illiquidity of housing for purposes of releasing equity.[9] Younger households, however, have benefited from the increased affordability of housing, and their prospects for accumulating equity in new homes purchased may be better than in recent years, when prices were inflated.

EXPLANATIONS FOR SAVING INADEQUACY

Analysts have offered a variety of explanations for why many people fail to save enough for retirement. One economic argument is that public policy has engendered moral hazard, so that many may look to government programs—Social Security, Medicare, and, in some cases, Medicaid—to take care of them after they retire (Gruber, 2009). Especially for lifetime low-income workers, support provided by such government programs can represent a significant percentage of income before retirement and also make it possible to mostly maintain the same lifestyle postretirement. Because Social Security is often presented as a publicly managed DB retirement program financed by lifetime worker contributions, many wrongly assume that there is no need for them to devote anything more to retirement saving. So while Social Security was initially conceived of as an insurance program (Scheiber and Shoven, 1999), survey evidence now suggests that many expect Social Security to provide everyone with a reasonable standard of living in retirement (Greenwald et al., 2010).[10]

Moreover, public policy in certain areas may have counteracted retirement policy. For example, when lifetime lower-income and middle-income households do save, they can find themselves subject to means-testing of Social Security payments (through the tax on benefits). Moreover, they may also be rendered ineligible for assistance through the Medicaid program as

---

[9]While the post-2008 decline in house prices has left many households with much lower housing equity than they expected to have, it is not clear whether this will translate into a major long-term macroeconomic effect. The committee does not believe there is evidence that housing's contribution to personal assets or consumption is changing because of the aging of the U.S. population. It recognizes that some have speculated that the value of housing will decline because of demographic-related shifts in household composition, but there is no clear evidence to allow forecasts of such a diminution of value.

[10]It is also possible that some Americans save little in the expectation that their children will take care of them. Many baby boomers have heavily invested in their children's education, and they may now be looking for that investment to pay off. Currently, much of the care received by the frail elderly population is informal, usually provided by adult daughters (Johnson, Toohey, and Wiener, 2007). Whether this will continue in the future, given the trend toward smaller and more split families, is unclear.

it encourages lower-income retirees to spend down what few assets they may have in order to qualify for benefits. Minimum-distribution requirements in DC plans limit retirees' tax deferrals and also discourage holding assets for late-life needs or deferred annuitization; these also can penalize "super saver" retirees.

Another potential factor contributing to low saving rates is financial illiteracy. That is, those who fail to understand basic economic and financial concepts may lack adequate tools for determining how—and how much—to save, as well as how to draw down assets in retirement. Studies have found that many Americans are financially illiterate, with a large percentage of households unfamiliar with the basic economic concepts necessary for making decisions about investing and saving. The problem is seen to be particularly acute among those who are most economically vulnerable, such as minorities, women, and those with the least education (Lusardi and Mitchell, 2007c and 2009). Not surprisingly, those who are least financially literate are also the least likely to be well-prepared financially for retirement (Lusardi and Mitchell, 2007b). More specifically, financially literate Americans are more likely to plan for their retirements, and planners are better prepared for retirements—with significantly higher wealth levels—than nonplanners (Lusardi and Mitchell, 2007a).

A related possibility is that people may underestimate their chances of living a long time in retirement, which might make them unlikely to save much for the latter portion of their lifetimes. But this idea is contested by Hurd and McGarry (1995), who conclude on the basis of subjective survival probabilities reported in the Health and Retirement Study that these probabilities correspond well with life table values and risk factors. In other words, it seems unlikely that overly pessimistic survival expectations are driving saving shortfalls.

CORRECTING RETIREMENT SAVING AND WEALTH SHORTFALLS

In view of the serious potential for retirement inadequacy, the committee explores next possible solutions to the problem. In particular, it focuses on what governments and employers might be able to do to help workers achieve retirement security, and what new financial products and services might help meet these deficiencies. Several approaches might be useful in correcting retirement saving and wealth inadequacies.

Boosting Saving

It is possible that more workers would save for retirement if there were universal access to employment-based retirement saving programs. Some have favored automatic enrollment of all workers, thus increasing program participation (Choi et al., 2002). Yet default saving rates in automatic-enrollment defined contribution plans tend to be set relatively low to encourage the low-paid to contribute. Others have proposed universal access to auto-enrollment 401(k)s or IRAs for employees of small firms, low-income workers, and workers who change jobs often, thus allowing more employees to take advantage of these programs (Iwry, 2004). Yet there is little agreement about how much more low-income households should save for retirement, because many already have difficulty financing subsistence consumption.

A different way to reduce the need for retirement income is to develop policies that encourage longer working lives and later retirement. For instance, raising the Social Security full retirement age and Medicare eligibility age would likely induce many individuals to extend their working lives, giving them additional years to make contributions to private retirement saving accounts as well as to the Social Security system. This could have the added benefit of reducing the number of years that they would need to be supported in retirement, though it might increase hardship on some and might also boost applications to the Disability Insurance program.[11]

Finally, making people more productive and likely to work—particularly in their later working lives—might help them get and hold better-paying jobs and thus increase the amounts they amass in retirement saving. Working in the other direction, if people respond to shortfalls by working longer, they might not have to save as much. In any event, encouraging later-life skill-building and training could make older adults more likely to get and hold better-paying jobs. An additional approach would be to encourage employers to invest more into wellness programs for workers, thus making it more likely that their workers will be able to work longer and live better in retirement as well as better understand and control health care costs.

Increasing Access to Retirement Assets

More diversification of the ways in which Americans provide for their retirement might also enhance retirement saving adequacy. One method already available is to allow older persons to take out reverse mortgages on

---

[11] Venti and Wise (2001, p. 27) argue that "the bulk of the dispersion in wealth at retirement results from the choice of some families to save while other similarly situated families choose to spend. For the most part, controlling for lifetime earnings, persons with little saving on the eve of retirement have simply chosen to save less and spend more over their lifetimes. It is particularly striking that some households with very low lifetime resources accumulate a great deal of wealth, and some households with very high lifetime resources accumulate little wealth . . . these saving disparities cannot be accounted for by adverse financial events, such as poor health, or by inheritances."

their homes (Mitchell et al., 2006). Reverse mortgages in many cases offer a reasonable way for people to access the equity in their homes while continuing to live there for the rest of their lives. Nevertheless, these mortgages are widely seen as expensive, and the decline in home values may make tapping into this asset less feasible for some retirees. Developing policies and regulations that improve the pricing and transparency of reverse mortgages could improve older Americans' retirement security.

Protecting Against Longevity Risk

As noted previously, an aging population may result in changes in the demand for various types of financial products. For example, there could be a shift from demand for life insurance toward demand for annuities. More generally, pressures to reform Social Security and the long-term shift in private retirement schemes from DB to DC plans of various sorts, as well as increased reliance on individual saving, imply that the financial risks associated with retirement income—asset returns and the stability and liquidity of assets—will increasingly be borne by individuals rather than public or private pension schemes. Such trends are widely expected to create significant demand for major innovations in financial instruments and markets geared to meet these varied needs. While longer lives are generally considered beneficial, they can lead to a "winner's curse" by increasing longevity risk—the chance of living so long that all retirement assets are depleted to support consumption. To protect against longevity risk, most financial advisers recommend converting a portion of retirement assets into annuities, which continue to pay as long as the insured party lives. While annuities play a critical role in theoretical models of retirement protection (Chai et al., 2011), in practice relatively few Americans buy them (Mitchell, Piggott, and Takayama, 2011). Public policy could make features and pricing of annuity products more transparent so that buyers could better understand them; this might enhance older Americans' confidence in annuities as protection against longevity risk. Evidence also suggests that workers with access to annuities through their workplace retirement plan are more likely to annuitize a portion of their retirement wealth at some point during retirement (Brown, Poterba, and Richardson, in press; Yakoboski, 2010). Public policies that encourage employers to offer annuities in their retirement plans would likely lead to more widespread adoption of annuities as one source of retirement income.

Some commentators have suggested that strong bequest motives might inhibit annuity purchase because people want to be sure that their heirs receive at least some of their retirement benefits in the event of an unexpected death. This concern would be valid if no current annuity products offered a "certainty period" as a provision in the annuity contract.[12] However, most annuity providers offer this provision in their product lines. Research by Brown, Poterba, and Richardson (in press) shows strong take-up of certainty periods by retirees who are starting a stream of annuity income. This evidence suggests that public policy should encourage annuity providers to offer products that include the option to purchase competitively priced certainty periods. Because long-lived individuals are also likely to have as many or more years of living with various diseases and disorders, it will be important to develop health-related products and services that provide for age-appropriate diversification of health care cost risk over the increasing length of older Americans' lifetimes. Better long-term care insurance products will be valuable here, including ways to provide for extended stays in retirement and nursing homes. Increasing availability and access to deferred annuity products that better meet retirement and estate planning needs would also enhance adequacy by providing better diversification of retirement risk burdens.

These broad issues pertinent to the level, stability, and liquidity of asset returns reflect various underlying specifics, many of which are expected to draw focused attention from the forces of financial innovation in coming decades. The most significant are likely to be longevity risk, duration risk, inflation risk, house price risk, health care cost risk, and of course the risk that markets for any or all of these risks may lose liquidity for short or even extended periods. The events of the recent financial crisis demonstrate graphically the potential for such disruptions to have major and potentially lasting impact on retirement income security for large segments of the population.

As yet, only scattered product or market developments have directly addressed aspects of this broad array of risks. A recent example is rapid growth in variable annuity products, which permit investors to pursue a broad range of asset accumulation strategies, followed by annuitization into a stable return stream. As large numbers of Americans approach and move into the traditional retirement ages, the committee expects to see the emergence of other products that address security of retirement income and management of longevity risks. This trend is likely to include more decumulation rather than accumulation products and development of markets to better price longevity risk and the duration risk associated with it. Considerable academic study in recent years, and by at least one private company, has focused on design of products and markets for management of longevity risk. Such products and markets offer the potential for greater flexibility

---

[12]A certainty period guarantees that the annuity will make payment for a minimum number of years.

for an individual asset holder or financial institution to take greater risk or lay risk off, depending on preferences and market conditions at any time.

Flexibility will be especially important for individuals as they take a greater share of these risks over their life spans. Some will wish to absorb more return or liquidity risk in the early stages of their life cycle in order to achieve higher long-term returns and shift to more certain, annuity-like return streams at later stages in their retirement. Provision of such flexibility to progressively larger portions of the population will require major developments in products, but especially in creating deep and robust markets for trading and managing the underlying risks. Because there appear to be many opportunities for new products in this area, policy makers might consider whether steps are needed to encourage new products and markets or to reduce disincentives.

Many studies have stressed the complexity and variability of behavior and demands in these areas from different segments of the population. For example, asset management practices vary widely by income and wealth level: The wealthiest accumulate assets in retirement, middle-income families decumulate financial assets in this stage, and lower segments of the distribution exhaust assets and depend on Social Security for retirement income. Several studies have noted the widening of income and wealth distributions in the United States and other developed countries, trends that are expected to continue and exacerbate the variability of retirement income approaches and needs across the wealth distribution in the future. These pressures may be felt especially at lower income levels, and hence on public pension schemes. More generally, trends in income and wealth distribution can be expected to heavily influence the mix of public and private mechanisms for both health care costs and general retirement income and so affect the patterns of demand for products and markets in which these risks can be managed.

A growing body of research shows the importance of financial literacy in Americans' ability to make effective decisions about retirement adequacy (Mitchell and Lusardi, 2011) (Box 7-2). Public policies that encourage employers to offer financial education, advice, and life planning (for all stages of a household's life) will enhance retirement security by reducing the errors associated with lack of financial literacy.

Most important, it will be critical to reform Social Security and Medicare so that future generations have confidence that these programs continue to be the foundation of our retirement system. Without reforms, the current financing shortfalls guarantee that the programs will be unable to continue helping Americans pay for their retirements, and since many Americans—including many of those who will be retiring in the next several decades—are relying on those programs for most or all of their retirement needs, their solvency is crucial to ensuring the adequacy of Americans' retirement provision. These government programs are particularly important for the longest-lived individuals as they are the most likely to outlast their personal retirement preparations.

IMPLICATIONS

This chapter has taken the perspective that already retired cohorts of retirees had the "wind at their backs," in that Social Security, Medicare, and generous corporate pensions enhanced their retirement security considerably. Moreover, the housing market provided excellent prospects for saving via their homes, and the stock market performed rather well until about 2000. The prospects confronting baby boomers are quite different: They face strong headwinds with regard to public program solvency, depressed housing market values, and lower and more variable capital market returns. And at the same time, longevity continues to rise, requiring either much more saving or longer working lives, or both.

Perhaps because of such changes, workers today are more pessimistic than at any time in the preceding two decades (Employee Benefit Research Institute, 2011b). And there remain important groups that face greater retirement insecurity than was true in the past. The lifetime poor are especially vulnerable; since they rely mainly on safety net programs, a humane goal might be to protect them from poverty as well as possible via government and charitable transfers. The more difficult question is how the middle class will fare in retirement. Some may be able to work longer and save more if encouraged to do so, and if they did, this could take some pressure off entitlement programs. Understanding this diversity in risk and saving profiles is key to the development of a better-integrated national retirement policy.

Moreover, population aging is likely to put increased pressure on household, employer, and government budgets, and in particular on the retirement savings component. The nation's fiscal imbalance is not driven only by aging, but aging and the financial crisis both have exacerbated these imbalances. In the absence of policy reforms and changes in household behavior, it is unlikely that Americans will do as well in retirement as they have in the past. Retirement insecurity and saving inadequacy are likely to increase rather than recede. To the extent that this inadequacy is due to people's financial illiteracy, early retirement, and reliance mainly on Social Security and Medicare, the problem of inadequate retirement saving is likely to worsen as the population ages.

Household savings adequacy will also depend on the cost of health care, which may prove to be even larger than out-of-pocket expenses if defined to include other costs related to poor health, such as moving expenses and the like (Poterba, Venti, and Wise, 2010). If population aging increases

> **BOX 7-2**
> **The Impact of Financial Literacy on Retirement Adequacy and Retirement Confidence**
>
> Prior research has concluded that financially literate individuals are more likely to plan for retirement, and in turn, to save effectively to that end. Yet a recent nationally representative study of young Americans found that a disturbingly high fraction of people aged 23-28 were unable to answer three simple questions about simple interest, inflation, and risk diversification (Lusardi, Mitchell, and Curto, 2010). The specific wording of the questions was as follows:
>
>> (1) Interest rate. Suppose you had $100 in a savings account and the interest rate was 2 percent per year. After 5 years, how much do you think you would have in the account if you left the money to grow: more than $102, exactly $102, or less than $102? {Do not know; refuse to answer}
>> (2) Inflation. Imagine that the interest rate on your savings account was 1 percent per year and inflation was 2 percent per year. After 1 year, would you be able to buy more than, exactly the same as, or less than today with the money in this account?
>> (3) Risk diversification. Do you think that the following statement is true or false? "Buying a single company stock usually provides a safer return than a stock mutual fund."
>
> Strikingly, one-fifth of the population could not provide a correct answer to the simple interest question; almost half did not understand inflation; and more than half did not understand risk diversification. Moreover, men were substantially better informed than women, and whites were more knowledgeable than blacks or Hispanics (Table 7-2-1).
>
> Low financial literacy will affect workers' and retirees' confidence in the retirement savings decisions they make and their ability to adjust to and recover from macroeco-

the incidence of individuals requiring long-term care (or nursing home) services, then these costs are another factor that will place tremendous strain on the resources of both aged Americans and their children.

Overall adequacy of retirement resources in this nation depends on the so-called three-legged stool: household provision, pensions, and sustainable Social Security and Medicare programs. Americans rely on all three systems to provide a well-diversified and adequate retirement portfolio generating sufficient assets to provide retirement security. Some argue that our prospects are bleak, given the current weakness of the job market, the ongoing volatility of capital markets, the underfunding of the workplace pension system, and the prospect of insolvency for Social Security and Medicare. Yet if government, employers, and private households are to successfully handle population aging, we must renew and strengthen the partnership to build retirement resources.

nomic shocks. For example, the Employee Benefit Research Institute (EBRI) 2011 Retirement Confidence Survey (RCS) found that workers are more pessimistic than at any time in the two decades the RCS has been conducted, but that retirees are not more pessimistic. The EBRI main report (p. 13) states: "The percentage of retirees who are very confident that they had done a good job of preparing for retirement fell from 39 percent in 2007 to 26 percent in 2008; it has remained steady since that time (31 percent in 2011)."

TABLE 7-2-1 Patterns of Responses to Financial Literacy Questions

Panel A: Distribution of Responses to Financial Literacy Questions (%)

	Correct	Incorrect	Don't Know
Interest rate	79.3	14.7	5.9
Inflation	54.0	30.4	15.4
Risk diversification	46.7	15.8	37.4

Panel B: Differences in Mean (%) by Respondent Characteristics

	Interest Rate	Inflation	Risk Diversification
Sex			
Male v. female	4.9	10.9	11.6
Race			
White v. black	3.4	18.7	12.3
White v. Hispanic	6.8	16.0	8.5

NOTE: All data in Panel B are significant at the 99 percent level.
SOURCE: Derived from Lusardi, Mitchell, and Curto (2010).

In short, U.S. population aging will result in a larger percentage of the population being of retirement age, as well as rising numbers of the oldest old. Nonetheless, these stresses are not insurmountable. These trends will require a number of new approaches to make sure that retirement savings are adequate for as large a percentage of the population as possible. In particular, public policies that encourage the development of new types of financial market products are needed to shift and pool risk more effectively than is done with current instruments.

Several other options exist for enhancing Americans' retirement security, including raising retirement ages, improving insurance protection and long-term care, fixing Social Security and Medicare, and instituting a number of private-market solutions: more saving, better financial literacy, reverse mortgages, and better long-term care and annuity products. It is also important to remember that uncertainty breeds fear and paralysis and makes it difficult for people to make decisions. The current situation threatens to reach the point where people are so fearful that they become paralyzed. Thus, doing nothing is not an option. Solutions do exist, and they must be implemented soon.

ATTACHMENT 7-1
MEASUREMENT ISSUES: NATIONAL INCOME AND PRODUCT ACCOUNTS SAVING AND INVESTMENT

In practice, there are many ways to measure saving and investment, a few of which are illustrated briefly here. These use national accounts measures, which are equal to income or output less depreciation, rather than balance sheet saving, which is the change in real net worth.

A conventional measure uses the standard BEA definition of saving and investment. This includes private and government saving as well as domestic and foreign investment, where domestic investment includes structures, equipment, change in inventories, and software. As the denominator, the committee uses net national product (NNP), which is the relevant measure of net income. This measure is called the conventional net saving rate and is shown in Figure 7-A-1 as "net S/NNP."

The National Income and Product Accounts (NIPA) personal saving rate (the fraction of personal income that is not consumed) has been criticized on a number of grounds, including the fact that it excludes capital gains (realized and unrealized). It does, however, include taxes on realized capital gains. NIPA does not include capital gains because the latter reflect a revaluation of the nation's existing capital stock and do not provide resources for financing investment that adds to the capital stock. However, many economists view capital gains as indicative of increases in the expected value of future output from existing enterprises. From that perspective, capital gains represent an increase in the stock of productive capital and should be included in savings measures.

A similar tension exists in the measurement of savings through pension funds. Employer contributions to pension funds as well as pension fund interest and dividend income do count as part of personal income and contribute to measured personal saving, but increases in the market value of assets held by pension funds, for example, are not counted. Proponents of this treatment argue that while an individual household can tap its wealth by selling assets to finance consumption or accumulate other assets, the sale of an existing asset merely transfers ownership; it does not generate new economic output. However, if asset appreciation represents a real increase in the value of productive resources available to society, excluding those gains understates the effective saving rate.

In any event, since the NIPA saving rate definition excludes capital

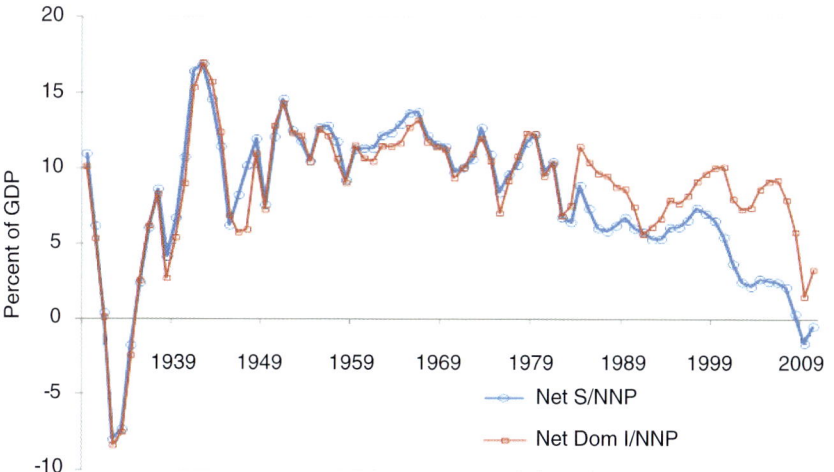

FIGURE 7-A-1 Net saving and investment using BEA definitions, 1929-2010.
SOURCE: Bureau of Economic Analysis (2011).

gains (as well as unrealized capital losses), it is likely to substantially overstate household asset accumulation in periods of rising asset values and may understate them in times of downward asset shocks. This mismeasurement problem is of particular concern for measuring the well-being of the aged in the United States, since over time more households have accumulated retirement assets in 401(k) accounts and IRAs. In other words, because those capital gains, when realized, will help cover expenses, they do represent a form of saving not currently captured by the NIPA definition. For this reason, some economists have argued that the NIPA definition does not accurately capture the true personal saving rate, so other factors should be taken into account.

Figure 7-A-1 also includes a different savings rate (net Dom I/NNP) using domestic investment for reference purposes. Standard national accounts treatment of investment is very narrow, most critically omitting most intangible investments as well as consumer durables. The conceptual definition of "investment" is that it is a use of output that increases consumption (broadly construed) in the future. Thus one can define "broad investment" as including all education, consumer durables, defense, research and development (R&D), transportation, and health expenditures of consumers and governments. There are different reasons for each, but the key is that they do not contribute to current enjoyment of goods and services (ice cream and concerts) but will enhance future enjoyment. Some do so directly by increasing productivity (as with education or R&D), while others are more indirect (such as military spending). Health is a complicated topic primarily because we do not have a good measure of depreciation.

Note as well that the calculations do not include a full set of accounts. This would require capitalizing each of the investments, estimating the depreciation rate, and then imputing income on the basis of an assumed rate of return. Note that R&D is scheduled to be included in the core national accounts in the next few years, and there are satellite accounts for education and health. National defense is a controversial topic, and in some of the earliest national accounts it was sometimes subtracted from both output and expenditure. Note also that this calculation excludes nonmarket income and output, which would be particularly important for health, where the benefits are largely nonmarket.

8

Capital Markets and Rates of Return

Population aging may affect the aggregate saving rate by raising the fraction of the population in age groups traditionally associated with the drawdown rather than the accumulation of savings. It may also affect the economy's average level of savings per capita, since individuals approaching, and shortly after, retirement age tend to have higher levels of savings than those at the start of their working career. The preceding chapter described both of these effects, which may affect the productive capacity of the economy. These effects may also, in turn, affect the rate of return that investors earn on their savings.

The average return on investments is a key determinant of the performance of funded retirement plans in both the private and public sectors. High rates of return enhance the power of private saving to provide for consumption and health needs in retirement. If investors can earn a real, net-of-tax return of 6 percent each year, for example, a dollar saved at age 53 will grow to 2 dollars at age 65. If the rate of return is 4 percent, however, a dollar must be saved at age 47 to double in value by age 65. With a return of only 2 percent, a dollar must be saved at age 30 to double by 65.

For many households, the ongoing shift from defined benefit (DB) to defined contribution (DC) plans has tightened the link between investment returns and retirement security. As discussed in Chapters 5 and 7, the returns earned by participants in DC plans, along with their contributions, determine their asset balances at retirement and directly affect postretirement living standards. In DB plans, the links between asset returns and participant benefits are weaker, since the firm or government offering the pension plan bears the risk of asset value fluctuations. When the assets in a private DB plan perform poorly, shareholders in the sponsoring firm earn lower returns because the firm must make compensatory contributions to fund the plan. Taxpayers play the role of shareholders in public sector DB plans. Past and projected rates of return are likely to affect the willingness of firms and government to continue DB plans, or at least continue them at the same level.

Private wealth accumulation supports a substantial share of retirement spending for some older households in the United States. For those households with substantial wealth, the rate of return can be an important determinant of retirement income. However, not all households have much exposure to financial markets, and many retirees have low levels of both financial and physical assets. For these households, rates of return are likely to be relatively unimportant influences on their financial circumstances.

Poterba, Venti, and Wise (2011) report that in 2008, the median holding of all financial assets, including those in individual retirement accounts and other similar vehicles, among households headed by someone aged 65-69 was $52,000. The analogous statistic was $112,000 for married couples. Because the ownership of assets is concentrated, average assets per capita are substantially greater than the assets of the median household. For households near the median as well as for those with fewer financial assets, their financial asset holdings are smaller than the value of prospective Social Security benefits. Financial assets are also smaller than accumulated home equity for those who own a home and smaller than DB pensions for those who are eligible for such benefits. Because the wealth distribution is highly skewed, however, there are also many households with substantial asset holdings for whom changes in rates of return are consequential.

Many factors affect capital market returns, including global demographic trends, long-run trajectories of productivity growth, investors' attitudes toward risk, and government tax and spending policies. Some analysts have suggested that population aging during the next few decades will drive down the general level of investment returns (Arnott and Chaves, 2011; Liu and Spiegel, 2011). They reason that as baby boomers approach the traditional age at which asset holdings peak, assets will be in plentiful supply and the equilibrium return on assets will decline. As *The Economist* reported (2006), some have even suggested that when baby boomers draw down their financial assets to pay for their retirement consumption, selling pressure may generate an asset market meltdown, a sharp decline in asset values. However, that scenario seems unlikely because it is inconsistent with forward-looking behavior on the part of financial market participants; it would require a sharp fall in asset prices in response to a predictable demographic event.

This chapter examines the ways in which prospective changes in the age structure of both the United States and the global population may affect rates of return. The increasing globalization of world capital markets requires a focus on how global population aging will affect the global supply and demand for savings and the rate of return available to savers (see Box 8-1 for basic terminology used in this chapter). The committee begins by presenting a general framework that highlights the various ways by which global population aging may affect rates of return. Because other factor inputs, notably labor input, also affect asset returns, the committee also explores how changing population age structure may affect labor supply and the decisions of young households with regard to human capital acquisition. Rising investment in human capital by younger workers can potentially offset some of the rate of return consequences associated with population aging, since the effective labor supply from a small cohort of highly skilled workers can be comparable to that from a larger cohort of less-skilled workers. In evaluating how population aging may affect rates of return, the committee draws on empirical studies that have compared rates of return in the United States and other nations to various measures of demographic structure as well as on findings from simulation models that have been calibrated to reflect central attributes of the U.S. and the global economy.

Demographic structure is only one of many influences on prospective rates of return. While the committee does not attempt to evaluate all the other forces that may affect such returns, it does note that the large fis-

---

BOX 8-1
Terminology

Throughout this chapter, a standard practice is followed and "savings" is used to denote a stock and "saving" to denote a flow. The stock of savings refers to the total amount of accumulated net assets that households, companies, and governments hold. The amount of saving in a given period, a flow, denotes the difference between income and consumption; the saving rate is the ratio of the flow of saving to the flow of income. An increase in the saving rate increases the supply of savings; an increase in desired consumption or investment increases the demand for savings. "Assets" can refer to any store of value, including physical assets such as land or plant and equipment, intangible assets such as patents, and financial assets that represent claims on the cash flows paid by companies, governments, or households. "Capital" here is used to denote the subset of assets that are used to produce goods and services. The capital-labor ratio, a common measure of the factor intensity of an economy, equals the ratio of the capital that is used in production to the amount of labor used in production. Labor in this context is a weighted sum, with the number of hours of labor input from different workers weighted by the workers' skill level.

cal deficits projected for the United States and other developed countries, which in turn are substantially affected by population aging, could play a significant role. These deficits will raise government liabilities and absorb savings that would otherwise be invested in productive capacity, leaving the economy with slower growth and fewer resources to support an older population. One consequence of the government-induced increase in the demand for savings could be higher rates of return. As is noted elsewhere, the lack of a credible strategy and its timely implementation for reducing projected deficits raises the risk of investors losing confidence in U.S. Treasury debt, which could lead to a rise in interest rates and a decline in the value of Treasury bonds.

HOW DEMOGRAPHIC CHANGE AFFECTS EXPECTED RATES OF RETURN: A FRAMEWORK

The balance between the supply of savings and the demand for savings determines the rate of return earned by investors. Households, businesses, and governments that accumulate savings hold financial claims such as bank deposits, corporate and government bonds, stocks, and deeds to houses and other real estate. Other households, businesses, and governments may demand savings to deploy in financing investment, personal consumption, or government consumption. They may issue financial claims, such as corporate bonds, to the suppliers of savers when they deploy these savings. An increase in the supply of savings lowers the expected rate of return to savers, whereas an increase in the demand for savings increases the return that savers can expect to earn. The decisions of savers about what share of current output to save each year, together with the value of savings that have been accumulated in past years, determine the aggregate supply of savings. The demand for savings, in turn, is determined by company decisions about how much capital to use in the production process, by government borrowing needs, and by household demand for credit.

An aging population can affect both the supply of and the demand for savings, and there are potentially countervailing effects. This makes it difficult to provide a clear-cut answer to the question, Are asset returns more likely to rise or to fall as a consequence of population aging? The committee concludes that the net effects of population aging on rates of return are likely to be modest.

This analysis is generally set in a framework in which global asset markets operate as an integrated whole, which means that assets can migrate freely to wherever they are expected to earn the highest rate of return. Migration of assets tends to equalize expected returns internationally: The global supply and demand for assets determines expected returns. This is why the aging of the global population, weighted by the amount of assets that residents of various nations hold, rather than the aging of the U.S. population, is most relevant for predicting how aging will affect rates of return. While the committee focuses on the mobile assets case, if asset mobility is limited, then while global population dynamics may affect rates of return, domestic demographic factors may also matter.

Table 8-1 shows the evolution of the U.S. old age dependency ratio, the global old age dependency ratio in which population aggregates are simply added up across nations, and a weighted old age dependency ratio in which each country's dependency ratio is weighted by its current and projected per capita gross domestic product (GDP) rather than its population in computing the global measure. The committee reports GDP-weighted values because it does not have detailed information on the aggregate asset holdings in each nation. The table shows that the global population today is older on a GDP-weighted basis than on an equal-weighted basis. It also shows that GDP weighting tends to reduce the disparity between the aging of the U.S. and the global population. The per capita GDP-weighted old age dependency ratio for the global economy rises more slowly than that for the United States for the next 20 years, but it catches up in the subsequent two decades.

Each year households decide how much to consume. When consumption exceeds their income, they must draw down savings to finance consumption, and vice versa. Companies decide whether to retain or distribute their earnings and how much to invest; and governments decide whether or not to save by collecting taxes in excess of current spending. Companies that seek resources to deploy plant or equipment in their business or to invest in new technology, households that wish to borrow because their desired consumption exceeds their current income, and governments that issue bonds because their tax revenues fall below their outlays determine the demand for savings.

TABLE 8-1 U.S. and Global Old-Age Dependency Ratios, 2010-2050

Year	U.S. Dependency Ratio	Global Dependency Ratio (Unweighted)	Global Dependency Ratio (Per Capita GDP Weighted)
2010	21.6	13.4	19.5
2020	28.3	16.1	22.7
2030	36.8	20.1	27.5
2040	39.0	24.5	33.9
2050	39.3	28.3	37.8

SOURCE: Donehower and Boe (2012).

Household Savings

The standard theory of consumer behavior has clear implications for the amount of savings that households will choose to hold. The theory posits that, all else equal, households prefer more consumption to less, smoother consumption to a more volatile consumption profile, consuming sooner to consuming later, and greater certainty about their consumption path. For a given level of expected returns, the desire to smooth consumption over time causes households to hold higher levels of savings when they expect consumption growth to be relatively slow; conversely they save less or try to borrow against future income when expected consumption growth is more rapid. Impatient households postpone the accumulation of savings until they near retirement age. Risk aversion motivates higher levels of savings as a buffer against adverse economic shocks. While the effect of higher expected rates of return on the household saving rate is theoretically ambiguous, under many reasonable modeling assumptions it seems that higher returns draw forth higher saving.

An aging population can affect aggregate savings in a variety of ways. Because older households on average hold more savings than younger households, an aging population will tend to display rising savings per capita. The desire to smooth consumption leads households to save while working so that they can draw down their assets to finance their retirement years. Higher aggregate savings per worker can affect the marginal product of capital—the amount of additional output that is produced from an incremental deployment of capital investment—if it translates into a higher level of capital per worker. Economic models of production imply that when the number of workers per unit of productive capital declines, the marginal product of capital will decline. A lower marginal product of capital would translate into a lower rate of return on incremental investments, which could reduce the incentive to save and partly offset the aging-related increase in savings per capita.

Population aging may also affect household savings by affecting the expected path of productivity growth and thereby consumption growth. Productivity growth is the most important determinant of consumption growth over long horizons. The rates of output and consumption growth over substantial periods of time are roughly proportional to the growth rate of output per unit of labor used in production. Chapter 6 reviews the evidence of the effects of an aging population on productivity and concludes that there is likely to be a negligible effect of the age composition of the labor force on the level of aggregate productivity over the next two decades.

Another way by which population aging may affect savings is its effect on economic uncertainty. For example, households may increase their savings if the imbalances between promised social insurance benefits and the tax revenues available to pay them create doubts about whether benefits will be fully paid or whether taxes will be sharply raised. Aggregate savings could fall, however, if developing countries introduce more extensive social insurance programs for their older citizens that reduce their incentives for private saving. China is currently pursuing policies of this type.

Savings by Companies and Governments

Companies and governments also make decisions that affect the aggregate supply of savings. Companies save when they retain earnings instead of paying them out to shareholders. Retained earnings generally are invested in a firm's own operations or in securities issued by other entities. Companies have a greater incentive to save when expected returns are higher and when there is more uncertainty about the availability of bank or investor financing. Because companies operate on behalf of the households that own them, household preferences are generally taken to be the fundamental determinants of company saving and investment decisions. The foregoing discussion of the effect of population aging on household savings therefore is suggestive of the forces that will indirectly affect corporate savings as well.

Governments save when current-year tax revenues exceed current-year spending, i.e., when they run budget surpluses. Often those surpluses are used to pay down government debt, but they also can be invested in real or financial assets. It is likely that increases in government saving are partially but not fully offset by reductions in household saving, so that government saving increases the overall supply of saving. The effect of government saving programs on household saving may depend on the nature of the tax and spending changes that are adopted. Except for a few years in the late 1990s, the U.S. federal government has been a dis-saver for most of the last three decades. Federal budget deficits have been particularly large as a result of the deep recession that began in 2007. Projections described elsewhere in this report suggest growing future deficits resulting from increased demands on social insurance programs.

Population Aging and the Demand for Savings

Companies use savings when they deploy various types of capital, such as land, real estate, equipment, and research and development capital, as inputs to production. They invest more when there are a greater number of profitable investment opportunities. When the return demanded by savers is low, a firm's discount rate will also be low, and the number of projects that will generate returns in excess of this threshold, or that will meet a present discounted value test, will be high. Population aging may affect a company's demand for savings in several ways. First, as per capita labor supply declines and labor becomes relatively scarce, firms may wish to substitute capital for labor; this would stimulate investment demand. More capital-intensive production processes may also allow older workers to extend their stay in the labor force. A mitigating effect is that raising the capital:labor ratio will reduce both the marginal product of capital and the return on capital investment, all else equal.

Households demand savings when they borrow to finance purchases of homes or cars, to invest in education, or to finance consumption. The aging of the population may affect household borrowing demand. Older households on average borrow less than younger ones—they are less likely to want to buy a bigger house or to attend college, and they have less future earning capacity to borrow against. However, if financial product innovations create new ways for older households to use their home equity to finance consumption, it is possible that borrowing by older households in the future may be higher than it is today.

Governments borrow not only to pay for current spending, but also to invest in capital that is used in the production of government services such as transportation, education, and health care. An aging population per se is unlikely to have a significant impact on that aspect of savings demand. A more important way in which aging may affect government demand for savings is by its impact on social insurance programs and associated budget deficits, as noted above.

Asset Market Equilibrium and Expected Returns

Expected rates of return shift over time so as to equalize the supply of and demand for savings. The foregoing discussion underscores the many factors that influence supply and demand and their interactions with an aging population. The underlying determination of returns, however, is straightforward. An increase in expected returns increases the reward to saving. Whether this raises or lowers the supply of saving is theoretically indeterminate and has proven difficult to measure empirically. At the same time, higher expected returns reduce the demand for savings, because it becomes more difficult to find investment opportunities that earn a sufficient return.

To summarize this discussion, Table 8-2 indicates the main channels through which an aging population can affect expected returns. Because the various effects point in different directions, evaluating the net effect of population aging on expected returns requires using an economic model that makes it possible to compare the quantitative effects of different influences.

TABLE 8-2 Some Effects of Aging on the Supply of and Demand for Savings

Aging Phenomenon	Effect
Link to supply of savings	
Older households have higher savings	Increases supply
Policy uncertainty raises precautionary savings	Increases supply
Higher capital-to-labor ratio lowers return to savers	Decreases supply
Productivity growth effects	Uncertain
Link to demand for savings	
Firms substitute capital for labor	Increases demand
Higher government deficits	Increases demand
Older households borrow less	Decreases demand
Productivity growth effects	Uncertain

RISK AND RETURN

The preceding discussion implicitly assumed a single rate of the return to investors, but in practice, there are a variety of real and financial assets with different risk attributes and correspondingly different expected returns. For example, households can save by holding stocks or bonds, or by accumulating equity in their homes. Earlier chapters of this volume examine how the choice between such alternatives may be affected by population aging.

From a macroeconomic perspective, a key question is to what extent an aging population will affect the aggregate risk appetite of the capital market. If older investors are more risk-averse than younger ones, then as the population ages, the price of risky assets may decline, and the required risk premium might rise, relative to historical experience. Several studies (notably Bodie, Merton, and Samuelson, 1992; Jagannathan and Kocherlakota, 1996) have suggested that older households may be less tolerant of investment risk because they cannot offset adverse shocks to the value of their asset holdings by increasing their labor supply. The typical advice of financial advisers to reduce exposure to investment risk with age is consistent with that reasoning.

Several recent analyses suggest that the link between age and the tolerance for investment risk—and its relation to labor income—may be more complicated. For example, Benzoni, Collin-Dufresne, and Goldstein (2007) argue that labor income is a significant source of long-run market risk for young people, and hence they would be expected to be more averse to investment risk than middle-aged households whose lifetime labor income is more certain. They predict a hump-shaped pattern of risky asset holding over the life cycle, which in aggregate would imply greater risk tolerance when a larger portion of the population is middle-aged. Changing tastes for housing and financial assets over the life cycle may also affect both the level of required returns and the risk premium for risky as opposed to safe financial assets. For example, Bakshi and Chen (1994) suggest that the demand for financial assets may increase as people age and their demand for housing diminishes; this could, in turn, affect financial market returns.

Empirical and Simulation Evidence on Demographic Structure and Rates of Return

To address the quantitative effect of population aging on rates of return, a number of studies have compared historical returns on financial assets in different time periods or different countries that were characterized by different population age structures. Other studies have used simulation models that incorporate the supply and demand elements that were described above to analyze the size of these effects. Each of these research strategies has strengths as well as weaknesses. Empirical analyses rest on relatively little historical experience with the type of population aging that many developed nations are about to undergo. Simulation modeling depends on many assumptions about difficult-to-measure parameters such as discount rates, the elasticities of substitution between consumption today and in the future, and the extent of openness in cross-country resource flows.

The committee noted in Chapter 2 that if age-specific asset holdings were not affected by population aging, the change in population age structure between 2010 and 2050 would result in a noticeable increase in per capita asset holdings in the United States. Table 8-3 shows mean net worth for households, classified by age of the household head, from the 2007 Survey of Consumer Finances. Because of the skewness of the wealth distribution, age-specific means are typically much greater than medians. For

TABLE 8-3 Household Net Worth by Age of Household Head, 2007

Age of Household Head	Mean Net Worth ($ thousands)
<35	106.0
35-44	325.6
45-54	661.2
55-64	935.8
65-74	1,015.2
>75	638.2

SOURCE: U.S. Census Bureau (2012, Table 721).

the 65-74 age group below, for example, the median is $239,400, compared with $1,015,200 for the mean. For analyzing the total supply of savings, however, it is appropriate to focus on means. If it is assumed that these age-specific means and household headship rates will remain constant for the next 40 years, average per capita net worth (all ages, in 2007 prices) would rise from $225,900 in 2012 to $248,100 in 2050. This increase of 9.8 percent would be attributable to the changing age structure of the population. If we just consider the population in the prime working ages 20-64, the ratio of net worth to population aged 20-64 will increase more rapidly (21 percent) during this period because the population aged 20-64 will grow more slowly than the total population in the coming decades.

Making projections of future asset holdings based on current age-related profiles is challenging, because it is impossible to fully disentangle age and cohort effects on wealth accumulation. For example, it is difficult to determine whether a decline in assets between ages 60-64 and 65-69 reflects a movement along an age-wealth profile, or the fact that those who were in the latter age group experienced different labor market and financial market conditions and were consequently less wealthy than their slightly younger counterparts. It is also important to recognize that the wealth distribution is highly skewed, so that average asset levels can be quite sensitive to the holdings of a small group of households.

There are also important age-related patterns in labor supply. The Bureau of Labor Statistics (2012) reports that the fraction of the population aged 18-19 that was employed in 2011 was 36.9 percent. The fraction rose to 60.8 percent for those 20-24 and to 73.8 percent for those 25-34. For those between the ages of 25 and 54, the average was 75.1 percent, with relatively little variation across age groups. After age 55, however, labor market activity begins to decline, with an employment:population ratio of 68.1 percent for those 55-59, 50.8 percent for those 60-64, and 16.7 percent for those over 65. The rise in the employment:population ratio in the intermediate age group is more pronounced for men than for women, who traditionally took time out of the labor force for child raising and who had a lower peak labor force participation rate. Age-related changes in the aggregate labor force could affect the rate of return on assets.

Empirical Analyses of Past Returns and Demographic Structure

Data on population age structure and rates of return, both over time in individual countries and across nations, can be used to examine the correlation between demographic factors and asset market returns. While several studies identify a strong relationship between a particular measure of demographic structure and a particular set of asset market returns, others find little or no association. The research has used a number of different measures of age structure, and some demographic measures do not seem to be related to return outcomes while others do.

Arnott and Chaves (2011), one of the latest studies in this tradition, examine the empirical relationship between population age structure and stock and bond returns in a number of developed countries. They allow for a relatively flexible relationship between age structure and returns and conclude that rapidly aging countries will experience substantially lower equity returns than other countries. The United States, however, is roughly in the middle of the country group that they study, with only modest return effects. Their analysis presumes that each country's demography is related to its asset returns, in contrast to the committee's focus on global aging as the key determinant of rates of return. Brooks (2006), in contrast, studies a number of nations and finds no robust relationship between age structure and asset returns. In fact, in countries with extensive stock market participation, such as Australia, Canada, New Zealand, the United Kingdom, and the United States, he finds that many households continue to accumulate assets well into old age. Poterba (2001) finds that measures of demographic structure have only a weak correlation with asset returns in the United States, with the strongest relationship observed between the price:earnings ratio and the share of the population in middle age. Geanakoplos, Magill, and Quinzii (2004) report that variation in the ratio of middle-aged to young households has predictive power for equity returns in the United States and several other nations. They also develop a simulation model that suggests a substantial decline in the price:earnings ratio for U.S. equities in the decades ahead.

The large variation of findings in the empirical literature is probably due to the relatively slow evolution of demographic variables in the recent past, which means that even when data are available for many years, there may be relatively little effective variation in the explanatory variables.

Simulation Evidence

The simulation literature on the effects of changing demographic structure has included studies of a single economy, best interpreted as representing the global economy with fully integrated capital markets, as well as studies that recognize the different current and prospective demographic structures of various regions of the global economy. Most studies consider a single asset category, which can be thought of as all capital invested in productive uses. The return on such an aggregate capital measure would correspond to a weighted average of the returns that investors earn on stocks and bonds issued by corporations and on their investments in owner-occupied housing and other real estate. The simulation studies suggest that there may be a modest decline in rates of return—between 30 and 100 basis points[1]—in response to population aging of the type that will take place in the United States and other developed nations in the next few decades.

A number of simulation studies have also considered how population aging may affect the equity premium—the difference between the expected return on risky assets such as corporate stocks and safe assets such as Treasury bills. Brooks (2004) suggests that when baby boomers retire, there will be an increase in the equity premium. This would translate into a decline in the value of corporate stocks and generate low returns for investors in this cohort. This result is driven by a large sell-off of equities by retiring baby boomers who want to hold less risky portfolios during retirement. Boersch-Supan, Ludwig, and Sommer (2007) reach the same conclusion. As with the effect of demographic change on overall returns, there is some disagreement about the potential effect of aging populations on the risk premium. Geanakoplos, Magill, and Quinzii (2004) and Brooks (2002) both predict a fall in the equity premium. Kuhle (2008) shows that whether the return on risky relative to less risky assets rises or falls depends on the relative price elasticities of the two asset classes. Existing empirical work does not provide definitive evidence on this elasticity.

FINANCIAL MARKET INTEGRATION AND CROSS-BORDER FINANCIAL FLOWS

The discussion so far has assumed that cross-border financial flows equalize the returns to assets invested in different nations. In such an integrated global financial market, when the aging population in one nation leads to a rising supply of savings and in the associated physical capital:labor ratio in that country, households can invest in other nations and take advantage of the lower capital:labor ratio elsewhere to earn a higher return than the one that would be available if the domestic economy was an isolated entity. If the population of a small, "open" economy grows old but the rest of the world has a stable age profile, there may be very little if any effect on the rate of return earned by its residents—by investing abroad, they can continue to earn the prevailing global rate of return. The open economy setting implies that rate-of-return effects may be small, but it also implies that there may be substantial cross-border financial flows in response to changing demographic structure. These flows may be of independent interest as a macroeconomic phenomenon.

This section describes the patterns of U.S. financial flows that could emerge over the next three decades in a fully integrated world economy. In addition, it highlights the potential importance of restrictions on financial

---

[1] A basis point is a unit of measure equal to 1/100th of a percent (i.e., 0.01 percent), often used to describe the percentage change in the value or rate of a financial instrument.

flows when different countries are aging at different rates. The evidence on how global population aging will affect financial flows is based on analysis of historical experience and calculations using simulation models. Bryant's (2006) analysis suggests that between the 1950s and the mid-1970s, demographic forces were a major factor behind flows of financial capital and direct investment from the Northern to the Southern Hemisphere. However, beginning in the 1970s, he finds that demographic change dampened, rather than augmented, these flows. His analysis suggests that the pattern of recent decades may persist for some time to come.

While the evidence on financial flows from simulation models is somewhat varied, several findings warrant attention. First, the paths of factor prices—the rate of return to capital and the wage rate—as well as aggregate variables such as assets, consumption, and investment, are considerably different under different assumptions about interregional financial flows. Attanasio, Kitao, and Violante (2007) and Boersch-Supan, Ludwig, and Winter (2006) find that population aging has significantly less influence on these macroeconomic variables in an open economy than in a closed economy. In these studies, developed-country wages increase less and rates of return decrease less under the open-economy than the closed-economy assumption. This affects the welfare of different generations differently, as shown by Krüger and Ludwig (2007) and Ludwig, Krüger, and Boersch-Supan (2007). Younger generations profit from the increase in wages, while older generations are likely to suffer from a modest decline in rates of return on assets. These patterns may be partly offset by government transfer programs that reallocate resources across age groups.

Financial flows have a moderating effect because they reduce the relative changes in capital:labor ratios. In these stylized models, initially, savings flow from fast-aging regions to the rest of the world, but this trend is reversed when households in aging economies start to draw down their saving. Yet these model-based predictions do not account for a number of other factors that may affect financial flows, and they also do not fit the recent experience of major financial flows from the developing world to developed nations like the United States. The recent experience underscores that other factors, such as cross-national differences in underlying saving rates, can play key roles. Prospective changes in social insurance programs in some developing nations could alter the demand for precautionary saving in those nations, thereby affecting their national saving patterns and financial flows.

Just as cross-border saving flows could play an important part in offsetting the impact of population aging in a given nation, cross-border labor flows could also matter. Immigrants tend to be younger than native populations, and if immigrant flows are large relative to existing populations, they could affect measures of the population age structure. The demographic projections that underlie our analysis incorporate forecasts of future immigrant flows to the United States. Since the United States is already at the high end of the developed world in its immigrant inflow, it seems unlikely that the rate of immigration will increase enough in the future to substantially alter the rate of population aging (see Chapter 3).

The comparisons between simulation analyses with and without open capital markets underscore the significance of capital controls and other factors that might affect cross-border financial flows in determining the effects of population aging on rates of return. At the moment, the United States is not experiencing financial outflows and is instead a destination for financial flows. The prospect of any restriction on outbound investments therefore does not seem like a near-term possibility. Over the longer term, however, if global economic conditions shift and developed nations with aging populations assume a larger role as asset suppliers, public policies that affect financial flows could matter.

An additional factor that may affect cross-border financial flows is the global pattern of debt:GDP ratios. The trend in this ratio is quite different in developing and developed nations. The International Monetary Fund (2011) observes that the debt:GDP ratio in emerging market economies has fallen since 2006 and is projected to fall further by 2016, while the analogous ratio in developed countries is rising sharply. For the world as a whole, the ratio of government debt to output is expected to change relatively little from 2006 to 2016.

"HUMAN CAPITAL DEEPENING": HOW MUCH OFFSET TO LABOR FORCE DECLINE?

The foregoing discussion of how population aging affects the labor force treated the age-specific pattern of labor market activity as fixed, even though there are a number of margins on which adjustment is possible. These include an increase in labor force participation at old and young ages, an increase in female labor force participation, which is still below male labor force participation in most developed nations, and an increase in the quality of labor through more training and education (human capital deepening). Increases in the global supply of labor, whether through expanded labor market participation or through increases in the effective per capita supply of labor, would tend to raise rates of return. The migration of labor from rural to urban economies in developing nations such as China and India is one of the important factors that may continue to influence the effective level of global labor supply.

Both physical and human capital serve to transfer wealth over time and even between generations. Savings and human capital accumulation are therefore closely linked. Worker investment in human capital is a factor that may attenuate the effects of population aging on asset returns. For example, if laborers are scarcer in an older society than in a younger one, and if young workers observe rising returns to supplying labor and take actions to enhance the value that they can deliver to an employer per hour of work, the resulting deepening of human capital will partly offset the rise in the capital:labor ratio and the associated change in the marginal product of physical capital.

Some broadening and deepening of the labor force is likely in response to the wage changes that will be associated with population aging. Such reactions are observed in simulation results from models calibrated to the U.S. economy. They show that increasing capital intensity as a consequence of aging will increase human capital investment, which in turn increases the productivity of physical capital. Ludwig, Schelkle, and Vogel (2010) find that the strength of that mechanism will depend, among other things, on the relationship between private investments in human capital and subsequent after-tax, net-of-transfer program returns.

It is also possible that changes in the labor markets of other nations, particularly those in the developing world, could affect the productivity of capital invested in the United States as well as the wages of U.S. workers. There are few, if any, quantitative studies of the cross-border effects of human capital accumulation. Because human capital levels across Organisation for Economic Co-operation and Development (OECD) countries are already high and rather homogeneous, spillover effects are probably small and they are likely to be difficult to measure. On the other hand, further human capital deepening in emerging countries can, and probably will, play a significant role in determining the capital:labor ratio of those countries.

The committee is not aware of any macroeconomic studies calibrated to developing nations, but it is possible to use microeconomic studies to assess the potential consequences of increases in educational attainment in these countries. Psacharopoulos and Patrinos (2002) report that the social return on an additional year of secondary schooling is about 10 percent in rich countries, 13 percent in middle-income countries, and almost 16 percent in poor countries. Private returns are even higher. Average years of schooling are 9.4 for rich countries, 8.2 for middle income countries, and 7.6 for poor countries. This suggests that in many nations, there is still room for improvement in human capital and for associated reductions in the capital:effective labor ratio. Such human capital deepening would raise the marginal physical product of capital.

As economically important developing nations that are well integrated with the global economy, such as China and India, embark on growth paths with rapidly growing educational attainment, they will play an increasingly important role in determining the global capital:labor ratio. Restuccia and Vandenbroucke (2011) present some evidence on prospective catch-up trajectories, suggesting that relatively rapid human capital deepening is possible in a number of developing nations. The trajectory of human capital acquisition in these nations will be a potentially important influence on the global rate of return to capital in the decades ahead.

Human capital investments in developing nations can moderate the decline in the rate of return available to U.S. investors as a result of global population aging. There are likely to be substantial differences across developing nations in the rate of human capital growth. In countries with relatively low birth rates and an aging population (e.g., China), the process of raising average human capital per worker by educating young workers can take a very long time. However, in countries such as India with rapid population growth and a large flow of young entrants to the labor force, raising the average education level in the population can take place over a shorter time period and potentially proceed for a longer time period.

HOUSING ASSETS

Much of the foregoing discussion treats assets as though they are competitively traded in an integrated world economy. While that might be an apt description of the markets for stocks and bonds, it does not apply to assets such as land or owner-occupied housing. Such housing, in particular, looms large on the balance sheets of older households in the United States. Poterba, Venti, and Wise (2011) report that for many older households, Social Security and owner-occupied housing are the primary sources of retirement security. Housing equity may provide an important source of financial support in response to adverse shocks. One of the first studies of demographic variation and asset prices (Mankiw and Weil, 1989) focused on how a shifting age structure might affect housing demand and ultimately house prices. That research suggested that an aging population would lead to lower housing demand and falling house prices.[2] While the two decades since that analysis have drawn attention to many other factors that may affect housing markets, a feature that distinguishes owner occupied housing from stocks, bonds, and many financial assets is that it must be owned domestically. This results in a tighter linkage between a nation's population age structure and the level of demand for such housing than, for example, between its age structure and the demand for corporate equity claims.

In nations with declining population numbers as well as aging populations, such as some countries in Europe, the demand for housing will

---

[2]The Mankiw and Weil analysis spurred considerable methodological discussion and critique in the 1990s (e.g., Hamilton, 1991; McFadden, 1994; Green and Hendershott, 1996) and continued to motivate research in subsequent decades (e.g., Federal Reserve Board of San Francisco, 2005; Takats, 2010).

decline in future decades. This will lead to a smaller total value of housing assets. This can occur through a decline in new construction, depreciation of the existing stock of housing, and/or a drop in the price of existing houses. The drop in house prices is a signal to builders to reduce the flow of new construction. Land prices are also likely to decline, since land, unlike residential structures, does not depreciate. The effects in the United States are likely to be more modest, because the U.S. population is projected to continue to grow through the next century. The effects on house and land prices are also likely to vary substantially across regions and even metropolitan areas.

CONCLUSIONS

Population aging in the United States, as well as global population aging more generally, is likely to have only a modest effect on rates of return. There is substantial uncertainty about the magnitude of this effect, as well as about the channels that will prove to generate the strongest effects. Some asset classes may be affected more than others. For example, owner-occupied housing in areas with rapidly aging populations may experience a decline in values, while land in the central business district of cities with rapid population inflows may rise in value. Cross-border capital flows and immigration could influence the ultimate effects. Moreover, there are close links between policies discussed elsewhere in this report, notably fiscal policy, and the long-run effect of population aging on rates of return.

There are important links between the financial markets in different nations, so the committee's focus for studying population aging and rates of return is on an integrated global economy. In considering how U.S. population aging may affect the rates of return available to U.S. investors, therefore, it is important to examine a number of features in the global economy such as the prospective growth rate of currently emerging economies and the degree to which immigrant labor can move from savings-poor to savings-rich nations. Given the uncertainties in the many forces that could strengthen or attenuate the effect of population aging on rates of return, the committee concludes that it is reasonable to assume that such an effect will be modest. It recognizes that financial markets in recent years have become more volatile, and its conclusion in part reflects the view that future volatility is likely to be dominated by nondemographic factors. If volatility remains high, this could affect the asset allocation choices of older households. It is important to recognize, however, that there are scenarios in which rate-of-return effects could be substantial and in which they would have significant effects on the retirement income of the future elderly population. Volatile financial markets may increasingly challenge older households with the need to make sound financial decisions.

ATTACHMENT 8-1
PHYSICAL RETURNS, ASSET PRICES, AND THE
TERM STRUCTURE OF FINANCIAL RETURNS

In a competitive financial market, the expected rate of return varies over time in a manner that equates the supply of, and demand for, savings. Savers directly invest in financial assets such as stocks and bonds that are issued by companies, they hold bonds issued by governments, and they also invest indirectly through financial institutions such as banks and mutual funds. Firms use the money raised from households and intermediaries to invest in physical assets—property, plant, and equipment—that are inputs into the production process. Over time, the income generated from such physical investments, net of expenses such as wages and maintenance, is used to pay interest and principal to bondholders and to pay dividends to stockholders or to repurchase their shares.

A simple example may help to illustrate the relationship between returns on financial assets, physical assets, and asset prices, and how those quantities are affected by the demand for and supply of savings. Consider a machine that produces $10 worth of output in excess of operating expenses every year forever. A firm finances the purchase of this machine by issuing a share of stock. The market value of the stock depends on the rate of return available to investors on similar investments. For example, if the expected rate of return is 5 percent over the next year and also for every year in the future on similar assets, then the price of the share would be $200. This is because the present value of a perpetual claim on X, discounted at r percent per year, is X/r. This price is consistent with the required return for investors: a 5 percent return on $200 is $10 per year.

If the cost of building another machine exceeded $200, no new machines would be produced because investors could make a higher return on alternative investments. Alternatively, if the production cost were less than $200, manufacturers would find unlimited demand for their products, since buyers could earn more than the 5 percent available on alternative investments. Thus, new machines would be put into production until the cost of building the units rose or the value of their output fell to the point where any additional machine built would earn 5 percent. Hence the forces of supply and demand for capital cause the expected return on any incremental unit of physical investment—the "marginal physical product of capital"—to equal the expected return on financial assets. The prices of existing financial and physical assets also adjust so that expected rates of return are equalized across investments. Those forces operate internationally; because investors seek the best investment opportunities at home and abroad, expected returns tend to be similar around the world. A more precise statement is that expected risk-adjusted returns are equalized; investments with higher levels of risk that cannot be reduced by diversification have higher expected returns than less risky investments. Tax differences across jurisdictions, and other market frictions, can also generate differences in rates of return across places.

The expected rate of return also depends on consumer preferences, which determine the supply of savings. When the aggregate supply of savings increases, for example because in an older society more people hold substantial retirement savings, the demand for existing assets rises. This puts upward pressure on asset prices and lowers expected returns, thereby encouraging greater investment in physical capital. In the foregoing example of a machine, if the expected rate of return were to fall unexpectedly from 5 percent to 4.5 percent, then the price of existing machines would immediately increase from $200 to $222 (= $10/.045). The higher price would encourage additional investment in new machines, which would continue until the cost of producing them rose or the value of their output fell to the point where the expected return on an incremental investment or the purchase of an existing machine was 4.5 percent.

Population aging is a predictable process that is unlikely to cause sudden changes in asset prices, but it may affect the time pattern of returns that investors expect to earn in the future. Investors may, for example, expect to earn different rates of return in different years. Continuing with the previous example, imagine that investors expect the rate of return on the machine to be 5 percent per year for the next 5 years, then to fall to 4.5 percent annually for the 5 years after that, and then to stay at 4 percent for the indefinite future, reflecting the higher amounts of per capita savings held by the older population at that time. The price of the machine would rise each year during the first 10 years, so that the sum of the $10 profit from the machine's production, plus the capital gain, would generate the return demanded by investors. It would reach $250 (= $10/.04) in year 10. Table 8-A-1 shows the price path that would provide investors with a total return—the combination of the $10 profit and the associated capital gain on owning the machine—that would equal their required return. In year 9, for example, when investors require a 4.5 percent return, the price would begin at $248.80, and the profit of $10, plus the $1.20 appreciation of the machine, would generate a return of 4.5 percent: [(10 + 1.20)/248.80 = .045]. Note that the price path rises gradually over time and levels off after year 10, at which point returns remain constant forever.

TABLE 8-A-1 Illustrative Price Path Needed to Provide Investors with Their Required Return

Elapsed Number of Years	Price of Machine (dollars)
0	234.88
1	236.62
2	238.45
3	240.37
4	242.39
5	244.51
6	245.52
7	246.56
8	247.66
9	248.80
10	250.00

9

The Outlook for Fiscal Policy

INTRODUCTION

Population aging will generate significant changes for the macroeconomy. As discussed in Chapter 2, barring significant changes in productivity growth, responding to population aging will require some combination of slower consumption growth and greater labor force participation, relative to an economy in which the age structure of the population is unchanged. Because the public sector finances a large share of the consumption of the elderly, population aging presents a particularly difficult challenge for government. Increases in life expectancy increase the number of beneficiaries of government programs, while declines in fertility lower the relative number of taxpayers upon whom these programs depend for financial support. Thus, as in the economy in general, population aging requires changes to government programs that ultimately involve some combination of lower consumption (which can be achieved through lower benefits or higher taxes) and higher labor force participation in order to remain financially viable. Furthermore, as explained in Chapter 3, the aging of the population is not a temporary phenomenon associated with the retirement of the baby boom generation. Rather, current projections suggest that the share of the population that is elderly is likely to remain elevated and even to increase over the foreseeable future. Thus, population aging is a phenomenon that needs to be addressed with changes to government programs.

The changing demographics affect both federal and state budgets. At the federal level, population aging raises expenditures on Social Security, Medicare, and Medicaid, while the projected slowdown in the growth rate of the labor force lowers payroll tax revenues and lowers gross domestic product (GDP) growth, making it more difficult to service existing debt. States finance part of Medicaid as well, so they, too, face financial pressure from demographic change. In addition, many states have promised pension and health benefits to their retirees, and these commitments will also put pressure on budgets as the population ages.

From an academic perspective, it would be interesting to distinguish the effects of demographic change from other factors affecting the fiscal outlook. However, in order to do so, it would be necessary to construct a counterfactual baseline (alternative scenario) of what the history and future of spending and tax revenues would have been in a world with no demographic change. Such a counterfactual is very difficult to create, because it is difficult to know how policies might have been different under alternative demographic patterns. To cite just a couple of examples: One would have to know how Medicare policies concerning payments to hospitals and physicians might have evolved differently in the absence of the looming fiscal challenges associated with an aging population or whether Medicaid benefits might have been more limited had states had to finance the education of the much larger cohort of children who would have been born had fertility not declined.

To the extent that the policies currently in place already reflect the actual or anticipated effects of demographic change, an examination of the current fiscal outlook may understate the impact of such change. For example, the 1983 Social Security Commission raised payroll taxes and increased the Social Security full retirement age. These measures reduced the imbalances in Social Security by, in essence, lowering consumption by workers through higher payroll taxes and a reduction in expected benefits. Thus, the current imbalances in the Social Security system provide a measure of how much further policy needs to adjust, but not of the entire effect of demographic change on consumption and/or labor force participation.[1]

On the other hand, for many parts of the budget, the projected imbalances between revenues and expenditures are only partially explained by demographic change. In particular, excess cost growth in health care and past tax and spending policies that contributed to today's outsized deficits

---

[1] Some observers believe that the buildup of surpluses in the Social Security trust fund was used to offset deficits in the on-budget accounts—that is, that taxes would have been higher or spending lower had those surpluses not been amassed. In that case, it is still true that the combined effects of the earlier tax increases and benefit cuts provide a good metric, when combined with the adjustments that still need to made, of the effects of aging on Social Security. However, if on-budget deficits are higher than they would have been in the absence of the tax increase, it means that, as a society, we have yet to make any of the adjustments required in the face of aging—some of the adjustments need to be made to shore up the Social Security trust fund, and other adjustments need to be made to pay off the extra debt that was amassed.

both contribute importantly to the difficult fiscal adjustments that will be necessary in years ahead.

Accordingly, it is difficult to isolate the effects of ongoing demographic change on the fiscal outlook. Furthermore, from a practical perspective, the ease with which our nation can adapt to the challenges of aging is greatly affected by the other factors shaping fiscal policy choices. For example, aging becomes a much more difficult problem in the face of rapidly rising health spending, and raising taxes to finance Social Security benefits becomes more difficult and has greater efficiency costs if taxes are already being raised to finance federal government debt or to pay for the pension and health benefits of state and local workers. Thus, in this chapter, the committee provides an overview of the financial imbalances projected for Social Security and Medicare, but it also focuses more broadly on the overall fiscal conditions of federal and state and local governments rather than solely on the challenges presented by aging.

FEDERAL GOVERNMENT

Social Security and Medicare are the two largest federal programs that support the elderly. In addition, Medicaid, a joint federal-state program that provides health care to those of modest means, is an important source of financing for the long-term care needs of the elderly. These three programs currently account for over 40 percent of all federal spending and almost 10 percent of our nation's gross domestic product. In addition, the federal government's publicly held debt now stands at roughly $10 trillion, or about 62 percent of GDP, and current projections suggest that, under reasonable (though still quite uncertain) policy assumptions, it will rise to 80 percent of GDP over the coming decade (Auerbach and Gale, 2012). The projected slowdown in the rate of labor force growth, by lowering the growth rate of the tax base, also makes that debt more difficult to service.

Social Security

The Social Security program assesses payroll taxes on workers and uses those revenues to provide cash benefits to retired workers and their dependents.[2] Thus, Social Security revenues depend on the size and productivity of the labor force, whereas Social Security outlays depend on the size of the elderly population. Both increases in life expectancy (which increase the size of the elderly population) and reductions in fertility (which eventually

---

[2]While payroll taxes provide most of Social Security's revenues, small amounts are also collected from the personal income taxes paid on Social Security benefits by upper-income taxpayers and from interest earned on trust fund reserves.

reduce the size of the labor force) contribute to imbalances in the Social Security program.

Figure 9-1 presents 2011 estimates from the Social Security Administration on the future of the program. Under the intermediate estimates, the retirement of the baby boom generation raises costs by about 25 percent, from almost 5 percent of GDP in 2010 to about 6 percent of GDP by 2030, while program revenues rise a little, on net, over this period.[3]

The traditional method used by the Social Security actuaries to portray the uncertainty in their analyses is to provide three alternative sets of assumptions: (1) the intermediate, baseline assumption; (2) a low-cost assumption, which assumes that life expectancy and unemployment are lower and fertility and productivity are higher than in the baseline case; and (3) a high-cost assumption, which makes the opposite assumptions. The actual outcome for future costs is very unlikely to be as extreme as either of the last two outcomes. According to the Social Security Trustees, these high- and low-cost projections correspond very closely to a 95 percent probability interval, meaning that there is only a 5 percent chance that the actual experience will be more extreme than represented by these two projections. Yet, even under these assumptions, the range of uncertainty is not that large over the next 20 years. For example, under the low-cost scenario, by 2030, Social Security expenditures will have increased only a little, to about 5.5 percent of GDP, while under the high-cost scenario, expenditures are closer to 7 percent of GDP. Revenues are fairly stable over this time period for both these scenarios.

Medicare

The Medicare program provides health insurance to Americans aged 65 and over, as well as to certain disabled Americans younger than 65. The Medicare program shares some features with Social Security. In particular, it finances a large share of elderly consumption, its benefits accrue predominantly to the elderly, and much of the financing comes from taxes on current workers.[4] However, the effect of aging on Medicare expenditures and revenues is more complicated than its effect on Social Security. Because Medicare provides health services rather than cash, the expenditures depend

---

[3]This chapter utilizes projections of spending from the Social Security and Medicare Trustees and from the Congressional Budget Office. These projections are based on different demographic assumptions than those presented in Chapter 3.

[4]According to the Congressional Budget Office (2011), in 2010 about 35 percent of Medicare spending was financed by the payroll tax, about 12 percent by beneficiaries' premiums, almost 40 percent through general revenues, and the remainder through various other sources, including income taxes on high-earning Social Security beneficiaries.

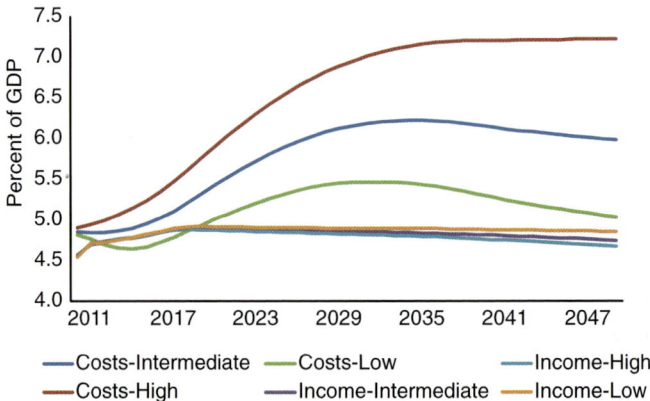

FIGURE 9-1 Projected costs and revenues for the Social Security Old-Age, Survivors, and Disability Insurance (OASDI) program, 2011-2050. SOURCE: Board of Trustees, Federal Old-Age and Survivors Insurance and Federal Disability Insurance Trust Funds (2011).

not only on how many people are eligible for the program, but also on their health needs and the costs of treatments.

One important question is the relationship between increased life expectancy and Medicare spending. Holding all else constant, an increase in longevity raises Medicare spending because it increases the size of the elderly population, and that increase is concentrated among the oldest old (those aged 85 and over), who generally have the greatest need for health services.[5] However, to the extent increased life expectancy is associated with better health at a given age, then Medicare expenditures need not rise as much. Indeed, several researchers have found that time until death is a better predictor of health expenditures than is age, and that taking this into account can lead to a substantial reduction in projected health expenditures (Shang and Goldman, 2007; Seshamani and Gray, 2004; Stearns and Norton, 2004; Lee and Miller, 2002; Cutler and Sheiner, 2001). However, much of this research uses data from the period when disability levels were still declining, and it remains an open question how the recent stabilization in old-age disability, discussed in Chapter 4, will affect future health expenditures.

A far more important source of uncertainty concerns the expected rate

---

[5] Increased life expectancy raises the share of the population that is 85 years and older, but the large flow of baby boomers entering into retirement raises the share of the young elderly. The average age of Medicare beneficiaries is projected to decline into the 2030s; after that, the average age of the elderly population increases gradually over time with increased life expectancy.

of growth of health spending holding health status constant. For more than four decades, health spending growth has exceeded GDP growth. As shown in Table 9-1, excess cost growth—defined as the difference between age-adjusted per capita health spending growth and per capita GDP growth—averaged 2 percent from 1975 to 2007 and 1.5 percent from 1990 to 2007. As a result, the share of health spending in GDP increased from 8 percent in 1975 to 16 percent in 2007.[6]

Most analysts believe that this rapid rise in spending in large part reflects the increasing value that our society has been placing on health care as we become richer, which has fueled the demand for new medical technologies and services (Smith, Newhouse, and Freeland, 2009). But health spending cannot continue to rise in excess of GDP forever, and it is likely that the growth in demand for health services will slow over time as expenditures on health increasingly crowd out spending on other goods and services.[7] However, there is little basis to predict by what means and at what rate that slowdown will occur. Many researchers believe that there is a considerable amount of inefficiency in our health system, and so part of the slowdown in spending could come from efficiency improvements. In addition, greater financial pressures on providers will likely lead to a slowdown in the rate of adoption of new technologies. The Congressional Budget Office (CBO) and the Centers for Medicare and Medicaid Services (CMS) both assume that excess cost growth in health spending will decline over time, although their assumptions about the rate of decline differ, particularly for Medicare.[8]

In the past, Medicare beneficiaries have received the same type of care from the same providers as those having other forms of insurance, and Medicare and other health spending have increased at similar rates (Table 9-1). However, the health reform measures enacted in 2010 (the Patient Protection and Affordable Care Act, as amended by the Health Care and Education Reconciliation Act of 2010, collectively known as the Affordable Care Act, or ACA) included provisions to lower the annual updates to provider payment rates and to cap annual Medicare growth. According to the 2011 Trustees' projections, with these payment changes, average excess cost growth for Medicare spending under the ACA will be close to zero over

---

[6]The share increased to 18 percent in 2009, but this sharp increase reflects the effects of the severe economic downturn, which lowered GDP more than it lowered health spending.

[7]When health spending is a small share of the budget, it can increase rapidly without having a large effect on other spending. As health spending becomes a larger and larger share of the budget, rapid rates of growth increasingly require large adjustments in the growth rate of other spending.

[8]In particular, the CBO assumes that, under a current law framework, the Medicare program will have less flexibility than states and private insurers to take measures to slow the rate of health spending, and thus that Medicare excess cost growth will not slow as much as that of private health spending.

TABLE 9-1 Excess Cost Growth (%) in Health Spending During Four Time Periods

	National Health Spending	Medicare	Medicaid	All Other
1975 to 2007	2.0	2.4	2.0	1.9
1980 to 2007	2.0	2.2	1.7	2.0
1985 to 2007	1.7	1.4	1.3	1.9
1990 to 2007	1.5	1.6	1.1	1.5

SOURCE: Congressional Budget Office (2011).

the long-run projection period; that is, most of the increase in Medicare spending in the Trustees baseline projection is the result of demographic change rather than health care cost growth.[9]

There is a great deal of uncertainty about whether these lower payment updates will allow Medicare beneficiaries to continue to be provided health care at a level roughly comparable to that received by the nonelderly and, if not, whether such a system would continue to be viewed as desirable (see Boards of Trustees, Federal Hospital Insurance and Federal Supplementary Medical Insurance Trust Funds, 2011, also referred to as the Medicare Trustees Report). For these reasons, both the CBO and CMS present alternative Medicare projections in which Medicare payments to providers are higher than those allowed under current law. The CBO assumes that the ACA cuts turn off in either 2020 (CBO baseline) or 2030 (CBO alternative), whereas the Medicare Trustees projections assume that the ACA cuts either last indefinitely (Trustees Current Law) or are phased out beginning in 2020 (Trustees Alternative). In addition, it is widely believed that Medicare's payment system for physicians, the Sustainable Growth Rate (SGR) system, will eventually be amended, as the administration and Congress have repeatedly stepped in to postpone the cuts to physician payments required under this system.[10] Both the CBO and the Trustees alternatives assume physician payments will be higher than those allowed by the SGR.

The impact of these varying assumptions, along with an estimate of how Medicare spending would rise under the assumption of no decline in excess cost growth, are depicted in Figure 9-2. Under the 2011 Trustees current-law projection, Medicare expenditure rises from 3.7 percent of

---

[9]The Trustees boosted their assumption about excess cost growth in their most recent report (Board of Trustees, Federal Old-Age and Survivors Insurance and Federal Disability Insurance Trust Funds, 2012), but aging is still the predominant factor contributing to the rise in the share of GDP allocated to Medicare over the long run.

[10]The SGR has annual caps on Medicare spending on physician and other services; when these caps are exceeded, the prices paid per service are lowered.

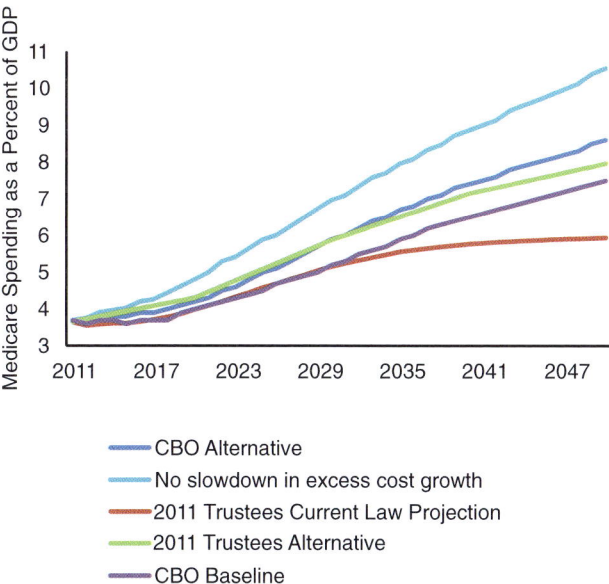

FIGURE 9-2 Alternative projections of Medicare spending, 2011-2050. SOURCE: Boards of Trustees, Federal Hospital Insurance and Federal Supplementary Medical Insurance Trust Funds (2011).

GDP in 2011 to 6 percent by 2050. Under the CBO alternative (which is similar to the Trustees alternative), Medicare spending in 2050 reaches 7.5 percent of GDP. The anticipated slowdown in health spending is important to these projections; under the assumption of no slowdown in excess cost growth, Medicare spending reaches over 10 percent of GDP by 2050.

Medicaid and Other Health Programs

Medicaid, a program that is financed in part by the federal government and in part by the states, is not an old-age program, yet it plays an important part in financing the long-term care needs of the elderly. In 2004, for example, Medicaid financed about one-third of long-term care services for the elderly (O'Brien, 2005), and in 2007 these services represented 14 percent of Medicaid expenditures (Centers for Medicare and Medicaid Services, 2011a). Table 9-2 shows the distribution of Medicaid spending by age in 2004. Per capita Medicaid spending is highest for those 75-84 and over 85, a reflection of the increased utilization and high cost of nursing home care.

TABLE 9-2 Medicaid Spending by Age, 2004

Age Group	Per Capita Medicaid Spending, 2004 ($)	Share of Medicaid Spending by Age Group (%)
0-18	819	24
19-44	662	27
45-54	737	11
55-64	1,026	11
65-74	1,112	8
75-84	2,058	10
85+	5,424	10

SOURCE: Centers for Medicare and Medicaid Services (2011b).

As noted in Chapter 3, increases in life expectancy are projected to significantly increase the share of people aged 85 and older. Thus, population aging may increase the demands on Medicaid. For example, assuming that relative Medicaid spending by age remains constant at the 2004 levels, projected changes in the age distribution of the population would raise Medicaid spending by about 10 percent by 2035 and 15 percent by 2050. Medicaid expenditure growth is also affected by excess cost growth in health spending (Table 9-1) as well by the recently enacted health reform, which expanded eligibility for the program. Taking into account the expected slowdown in health spending growth, the aging of the population, and the effects of the recently enacted health reform, the CBO projects (Figure 9-3) that federal spending for Medicaid and other non-Medicare health programs (the much smaller Children's Health Insurance program

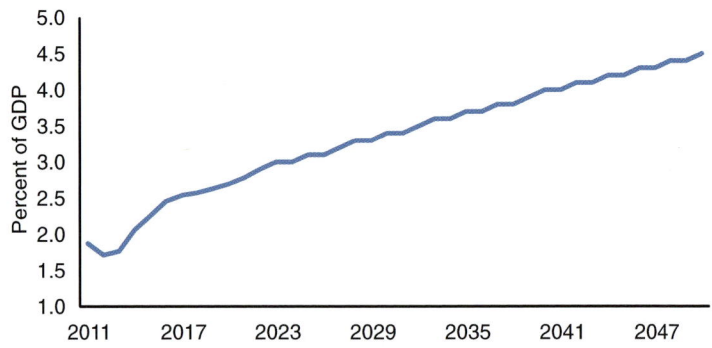

FIGURE 9-3 Projected federal spending on Medicaid and other health programs, 2011-2050. SOURCE: Congressional Budget Office (2011, Underlying Tables, Table B-1, Extended Baseline).

and the future outlays for health insurance subsidies under health reform) will rise from about 2 percent of GDP in 2011 to 3.7 percent in 2035 and 4.5 percent in 2050.[11]

STATE AND LOCAL GOVERNMENT

For the state and local sector, there are likely to be two significant sources of fiscal pressure going forward. First, since states finance roughly 40 percent of Medicaid spending, on average, rapid increases in Medicaid expenditures are also likely to put pressure on state budgets as well. Second, although states are subject to balanced budget requirements in their operating funds and so typically don't have substantial amounts of debt outstanding, they do have implicit debt in the form of unfunded liabilities for the pension and retiree health benefits of state workers (Munnell et al., 2011).

There has been much less attention paid to long-term budget projections for the state and local sector than to the federal government sector. One exception is the Government Accountability Office (GAO), which reports its projections for state and local expenditures and revenues through 2060 (Government Accountability Office, 2012). The GAO examines both the impact of health care cost growth and the liabilities for state and local pension and retiree health benefits, assuming that these benefits are fully paid as scheduled. According to these projections, without policy changes, state and local government operating budgets are likely to be under increasing stress over time. By 2025, for example, the GAO's base case shows an imbalance between revenues and expenditures of about 1.5 percent of GDP, rising to close to 4 percent of GDP by 2060. Much of this rise is attributable to rapidly increasing excess cost growth (the GAO assumes slightly faster growth of excess health cost growth for Medicaid and retiree health insurance than does the CBO). While not strictly comparable to the CBO projections, the GAO projections show that, even with the assumed slowdown in health spending, expenditure and revenue adjustments will need to be made in the state and local sector as well. While not all of these adjustments are directly attributable to demographic change, they are an important component of the overall fiscal outlook for the U.S. economy.

---

[11] Medicaid is by far the largest component of these. For example, in 2021, under the CBO projections, Medicaid accounts for 83 percent of the federal government spending on health programs other than Medicare. The CBO assumes that excess cost growth in these health programs will decline linearly over time, from 1.7 percentage points per year in 2022 to 0 in 2086.

PUTTING THE PIECES TOGETHER: THE LONG-TERM BUDGET OUTLOOK

The sustainability of federal fiscal policy is affected not only by the expected growth in entitlement programs but also by the current level of national debt and by the expected trajectories for tax revenues and discretionary spending. Auerbach and Gale (2012) present a detailed analysis of alternative trajectories of total federal spending, revenues, and debt under a variety of assumptions about fiscal policy.

Figure 9-4 presents two such scenarios for noninterest expenditure and revenues. The more optimistic scenario uses the Medicare Trustees projections for Medicare spending and assumes that taxes will rise to about 21 percent of GDP over the long term, 3 percentage points above the 18 percent average recorded from 1970 to 2007. In addition, it assumes that savings from the Budget Control Act of 2011 will materialize. The more pessimistic scenario uses the CBO "alternative" projection for Medicare spending, which is considerably higher than that of the Medicare Trustees, assumes that Congress will maintain tax revenues at roughly its recent historical average of 18 percent of GDP, and assumes that parts of the Budget Control Act will be repealed.[12] This scenario can be interpreted as one in which taxes and entitlement programs operate largely as they have in the past, whereas the optimistic scenario already incorporates some adjustments to demographic change, including a reining in of health care cost growth and an increase in average tax rates.

Under the optimistic scenario, noninterest expenditures fall from 22 percent to roughly 20 percent of GDP by 2018 as the economy recovers and then rise slowly thereafter, to about 22 percent by 2030 and 23 percent by 2050. Under the more pessimistic scenario, noninterest outlays rise faster, reaching almost 26 percent by 2050. With tax revenues of 21 percent and 18 percent of GDP, respectively, the primary deficit (that is, the deficit excluding interest payments on the national debt) reaches 2 percent of GDP by 2050 under the optimistic scenario and almost 8 percent in the pessimistic scenario.

Figure 9-5 shows the deficit projections implied by these two sets of expenditure and revenue projections, including projected interest payments. In both scenarios, the deficit declines sharply over the next few years relative to GDP as the economy recovers, and then begins to climb. In the optimistic scenario, the deficit falls to close to 1 percent of GDP over the next decade and then increases only gradually over time, reaching 4 percent of GDP by 2030 and almost 8 percent of GDP by 2050. Even under this positive sce-

---

[12] In particular, the pessimistic scenario assumes that the $1.2 trillion in budget savings that would be triggered by automatic sequestration under the Budget Control Act of 2011 will be repealed.

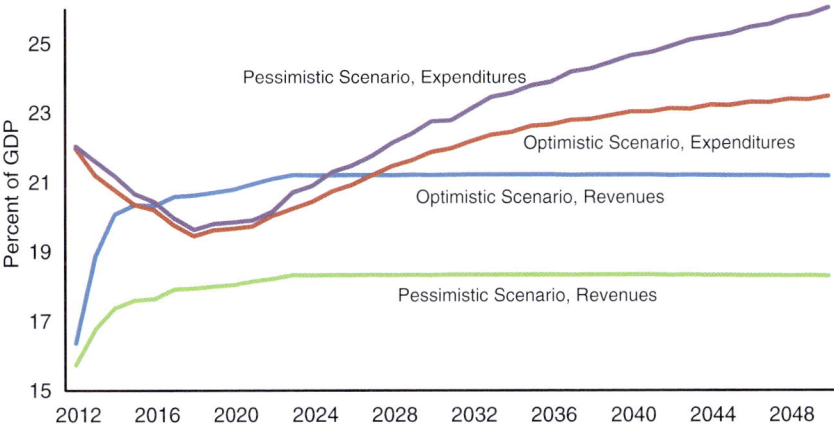

FIGURE 9-4 Alternative federal projections of revenue and noninterest outlays, 2012-2050. SOURCE: Auerbach and Gale (2012).

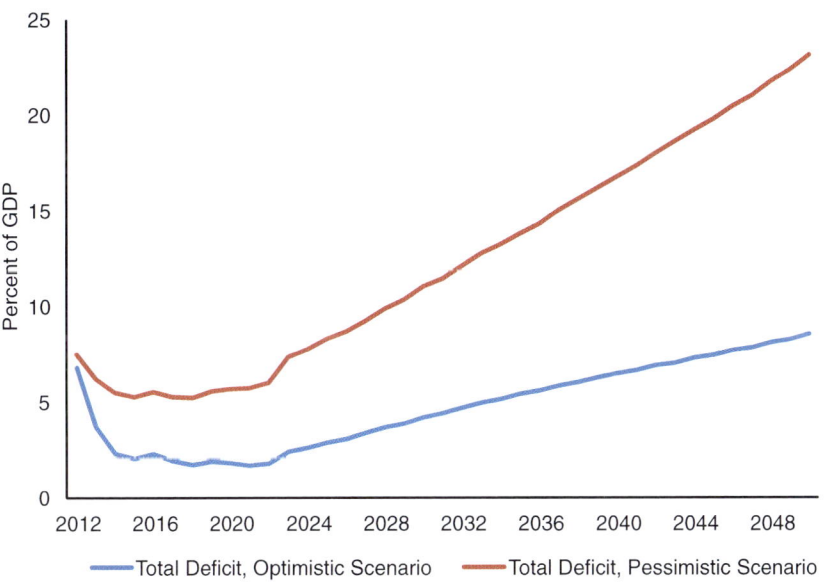

FIGURE 9-5 Alternative federal deficit projections, 2012-2050. SOURCE: Committee calculations based on Auerbach and Gale (2012).

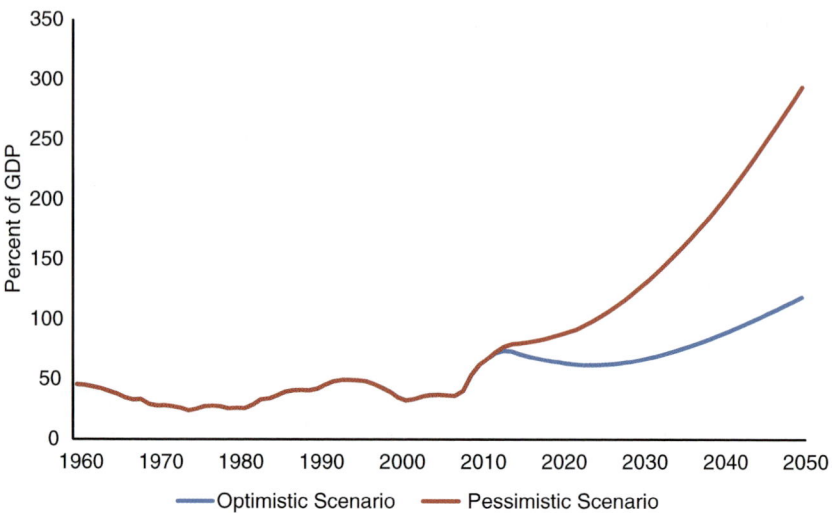

FIGURE 9-6 Alternative federal debt:GDP ratios, 2012-2050. SOURCE: Committee calculations based on Auerbach and Gale (2012).

nario, future adjustments will still be necessary. In the pessimistic scenario, the deficit hovers around 5 percent of GDP for much for the next decade but climbs sharply thereafter, reaching over 10 percent of GDP by 2030 and over 20 percent of GDP by 2050. The sharp acceleration in the future deficits under the pessimistic scenario reflects the combination of continued rapid growth in health expenditures as well as rapidly rising interest payments from continued large deficits.

Figure 9-6 shows the implied debt:GDP ratios under these two sets of projections. Under the most optimistic set of assumptions, the debt:GDP ratio falls over the next 15 years and then begins to climb sharply, reaching 100 percent of GDP by 2046. Under the more pessimistic set of projections, the debt:GDP ratio climbs much more rapidly, reaching 100 percent of GDP by 2027 and 200 percent of GDP by 2043.

The debt:GDP ratio cannot continue to rise indefinitely; at some point, investors would become uncertain of full repayment (or worry about repayment in greatly inflated dollars) and start demanding a risk premium[13] on U.S. Treasury securities. At that point, rising interest payments on the debt would trigger even larger deficits, potentially resulting in an unsustainable deficit spiral. Although there is uncertainty as to exactly what level of debt

---

[13] The extra expected return over the risk-free rate demanded by investors to compensate for the volatility of returns or the possibility of default of risky assets.

TABLE 9-3 Adjustment Needed to Maintain the 2011 Debt/GDP Ratio Through 2050

	Required Adjustment (% of GDP)	
Adjustment Takes Place in	Optimistic Scenario	Pessimistic Scenario
2012	1.1	4.8
2022	1.7	6.1
2032	2.4	7.7

SOURCE: Committee calculations based on Auerbach and Gale (2012).

will elicit such a reaction, it is clear that fiscal policy adjustments will need to be made eventually. In particular, even through 2050, it is unlikely that the pessimistic scenario could actually unfold, as it is unlikely that investors would be willing to continue to finance the projected deficits.

One response to population aging would be to attempt to smooth the required adjustments over time in order to minimize the size of the adjustment in any given year. Because population aging is projected to be permanent, however, spreading the adjustments equally over time would require the government to build up a large stock of assets and to use the earnings on those assets to help finance part of future government spending. Alternatively, the government could smooth through the adjustments over a more finite period. For example, Table 9-3 presents calculations based on Auerbach and Gale (2012) showing the size of the adjustments required in order for the debt:GDP ratio in 2050 to be the same as it was in 2011. For example, under the more optimistic scenario, which already includes higher revenues and lower health spending growth than the historical averages, an immediate and permanent change to tax revenues or expenditures equal to just over 1 percent of GDP would leave the debt:GDP ratio in 2050 the same as it is today; under this scenario, the debt:GDP ratio would decline to 44 percent over roughly the next two decades years, and then it would start to climb again, reaching 68 percent in 2050. Alternatively, if the adjustment were delayed until 2022, a 1.7 percent of GDP adjustment would be required, and if it were delayed until 2032, a 2.4 percent of GDP reduction in expenditures or increase in taxes would be required. Under the pessimistic scenario, which assumes significantly lower tax revenues and higher health expenditures, the required adjustments are significantly larger.

MACROECONOMIC IMPLICATIONS OF RESPONSES TO DEMOGRAPHIC CHANGE

The aforementioned budget projections indicate that a large change in the combined trajectory of federal tax revenues and expenditures will be required over the coming decades. These changes will have important macroeconomic consequences, but there is no natural baseline against which to measure these macroeconomic effects because the status quo trajectory is not a feasible one—it would lead to an exploding and unsustainable level of national debt. Thus, we can only compare the effects of different feasible paths, especially their relative effects on capital accumulation and labor supply, both in the aggregate and across generations. To estimate these effects, several attributes of budget adjustments will be relevant, including those described in the next seven subsections.

How Quickly the Changes Are Implemented

Under both the optimistic and pessimistic scenarios, annual deficits are projected to grow over time as a share of GDP, even when debt service costs are excluded. Thus, as mentioned above, if the adjustment process targets the rate of debt accumulation, the magnitude of deficit cuts will grow over time as a share of GDP.

A different policy that would lessen the magnitude of the required deficit cuts over time would be to make larger immediate adjustments to taxes and spending policies that could temporarily lower the debt:GDP ratio. This would have the effect of smoothing the adjustments across more cohorts. However, it is unclear how much of this type of "prefunding" is feasible. According to Auerbach (2002 and 2003), there is a predictable reaction function of government spending to the deficit: As the deficit falls as a share of GDP, government spending increases and tax revenues fall as a share of GDP. Thus, policies that would significantly lower deficits ahead of the baby boom retirement, while possibly economically attractive, might prove politically unsustainable.

On the other hand, waiting too long to announce and implement policy changes is a risky strategy. As noted above, it is impossible to predict the level of debt at which investors might lose confidence in the ability or willingness of the United States to fully repay its debts. This loss of confidence could occur quite suddenly, and it might lead to a period of financial crisis or a situation in which policy adjustments would have to be quite large and immediate, which could have deleterious effects on short-term macroeconomic performance (National Research Council and National Academy of Public Administration, 2010).

When Changes Are Announced or Anticipated

Changes that are implemented in the future may nonetheless be announced or anticipated many years before. If announcements of future policies are credible or if expectations reflect an accurate assessment of the policies that eventually will be undertaken, then these policies can affect behavior long before their implementation. An example is the phased increase in the Social Security full retirement age, which was enacted in 1983 but implemented over a long period beginning several years after enactment. To the extent individuals are forward looking, this change in policy would have boosted private saving in the years prior to its implementation, as people increased their saving in anticipation of lower future Social Security benefits.

Changes That Explicitly or Implicitly Increase Marginal Tax Rates

Some policy changes quite explicitly increase marginal tax rates.[14] Most tax increases would do so, unless accompanied by changes in tax structure. But many marginal tax rates are implicit, as in the case of the means-testing of social insurance benefits. This point has been made quite frequently in the context of antipoverty programs, where the simultaneous loss of different benefits for those who enter work can in combination lead to very high marginal tax rates and create a poverty "trap" that strongly discourages exits from poverty and dependence. But the point also applies to universal old-age entitlement programs. For example, the share of Social Security benefits subject to the income tax depends on retirees' other income, which imposes an implicit marginal tax rate (in addition to the explicit one) on that other income. Similarly Medicare Part B premiums are now income-based, which also imposes a tax on such income.

Note that implicit marginal tax rates on income may be imposed through the tax system (as in the case of Social Security benefit taxation) or through the expenditure system (as in the case of Medicare premiums, which are classified in the budget as offsetting receipts that reduce expenditures). This fact highlights an important point: Macroeconomic effects will depend on the distribution and structure of budget changes but not directly on whether these changes are recorded on the tax side or the expenditure side. Though this distinction sometimes appears paramount in political discussions, it is of little relevance for economic analysis except to the extent that the underlying behavioral effects of tax or expenditure changes may systematically differ.

The Intergenerational Distribution of Policy Changes

The intergenerational distribution of policy changes will relate to the first point above, because changes that are delayed are likely to affect

---

[14]The marginal tax rate is the rate that would have to be paid on any additional taxable income earned, which may be higher than the rate paid without additional earnings.

younger generations. But two policies of the same magnitude implemented at the same time may have different distributional effects among generations. For example, an immediate, permanent cut in Social Security benefits will affect older generations more than an immediate, permanent increase in Social Security taxes with the same budget result. Similarly, a consumption tax would affect older generations more than an increase in the income tax. The generational distribution of deficit reductions will matter for aggregate economic activity because generations have different propensities to consume goods and leisure out of income changes, and they are affected differently by changes in marginal tax rates. For example, we would expect larger reductions in consumption (say, through reductions in tax exemptions) from income reductions imposed on 70-year-olds than from equal-size reductions imposed on 40-year-olds, because the latter group is in a better position to offset income losses by increasing labor force participation. Likewise, we would expect larger changes in labor supply from increased marginal income tax rates on 40-year-olds than from increased marginal income tax rates on 70-year-olds, who are mostly retired and out of the labor force.

The distributional effects of a program of budget adjustments over time can be summarized using generational accounts, which cumulate the effects on different generations at different dates. Such accounts, however, focus on incidence and hence must be complemented by analysis of how changes in incentives, via marginal tax rates, are distributed across generations and, as discussed next, within generations. Also, because generational accounts are forward-looking calculations, their usefulness for macroeconomic analysis hinges on the extent to which the affected individuals (1) actually are forward looking and (2) are not liquidity-constrained[15] in a manner that makes future taxes and benefits irrelevant, as they would be for households with little or no saving who spend essentially all of their disposable income each year.

The Intragenerational Distribution of Policy Changes

Two policies with the same timing, intergenerational distribution, and marginal tax rate changes can affect members of a given cohort differently. For example, one might vary the progressivity of a given cut in Social Security benefits. As with differences across generations, differences in the impact of deficit cuts within a generation can be expected to have different effects on labor supply and saving. For example, lower-income individuals are more likely to be liquidity-constrained and hence to suffer a big-

---

[15]That is, without sufficient cash to make purchases, and/or unable to borrow to consume or invest.

ger decline in consumption in response to a given reduction in after-tax income. Also, those who are liquidity-constrained or myopic are less likely to respond to anticipated future policy changes; such individuals may not change their labor force or saving behavior, which become irrelevant when current decisions are constrained.

The Timing of Tax Increases and Benefit Cuts over a Lifetime

One of the important rationales for the existence of programs like Social Security and Medicare is that many people are not farsighted enough to adequately save for retirement, and these programs are a form of forced saving, at least from the individual's standpoint. Thus, while people with perfect foresight will adjust their consumption optimally in response to an announced cut in benefits, many others may not. This means that, even for an individual, a tax increase and benefit cut that lower lifetime resources by the same amount can have different effects, with changes occurring in the distant future possibly having a smaller impact today.

The Role That Policy Changes Play in Insuring or Exacerbating Risk

Under reasonable assumptions, uncertainty about future resources affects current behavior. Individuals may engage in precautionary saving if the future is uncertain, and they may also work more or delay retirement. These effects are in addition to those resulting from expected changes in resources. Uncertainty is always present in the economy, and indeed one stated purpose of social insurance is to reduce such uncertainty by cushioning the shocks of economic forces on particular individuals or, through intergenerational risk-sharing, entire cohorts. But uncertainty about future policy changes might exacerbate existing uncertainty. For example, budget deficits rise when the economy is weak because of a loss in revenues, so if policy aims to achieve a fixed budget reduction, budget cuts must be larger when the economy is weak and individual resources are low.

In summary, to analyze the macroeconomic effects of a given policy trajectory, one would like to estimate the inter- and intragenerational distribution of changes in resources and marginal tax rates under the policy, the dates at which future policy changes are anticipated, and the distribution of possible policy paths and how these paths relate to the economy's possible trajectories. Sophisticated general equilibrium models with overlapping generations, forward-looking agents, and within-generation heterogeneity do exist, but it would be a considerable challenge to construct a detailed model that incorporates realistic tax and expenditure elements and is capable of taking all of the factors discussed into account simultaneously. Thus, the most reasonable approach is to use different models designed to capture different elements of the overall picture, simplifying where possible to keep the most important elements of particular policy changes in focus.

To see how these different channels of transmission from policy to the economy may operate, it is helpful to focus on the three broad categories of policy adjustments that have been considered to address the fiscal imbalances.

Steps to Rein in Excess Health Care Cost Growth

One of the key differences between the most optimistic and most pessimistic scenarios in Figure 9-4 is the assumption about the trajectory of federal spending on health programs after 2020. Under the optimistic scenario, per-beneficiary health spending grows roughly in line with GDP, whereas under the pessimistic scenario, rapid health spending is responsible for a large and growing portion of the fiscal imbalances over time.

Accordingly, measures like the ACA that attempt to lower the overall health spending of the elderly are likely to be an important component of long-term fiscal policy. Yet the macroeconomic consequences of such measures are among the most difficult to determine. If, as some believe, changes in Medicare policy can induce innovations in health care delivery that lead to reduced spending without a reduction in the quality of care (for example, by eliminating duplication of services, eliminating unnecessary care, or reducing costly errors), then these policy changes would help address the fiscal problem without any required reduction in living standards. On the other hand, lowering the rate of growth of health spending may be accompanied by reduced access to care and a slower rate of growth of innovation, which would lower the living standards of the elderly relative to a baseline in which spending continued to rise faster than GDP. Finally, cuts in Medicare spending could lead to lower income for health service providers, which would be equivalent to a tax on providers. Over time, such a tax could reduce the attractiveness of practicing medicine, which could lead to lower quality and reduced access as well.

Benefit Cuts

There is a wide variety of policies that could lower the growth rate of entitlement spending beyond changing the growth rate of health care costs. Such options include changing the age of eligibility for benefits, changing the generosity of benefits, and limiting benefit growth by increased reliance on means-testing. These different approaches would likely have different distributional consequences; in addition, they might also have differential effects on labor supply.

For example, a policy to index retirement ages (particularly the full retirement age) for Social Security benefits to life expectancy would lower benefits disproportionately for those with a shorter life expectancy. Given the dramatic widening of the gap in life expectancies across the income distribution seen in recent decades (Congressional Budget Office, 2008), this distributional effect might be deemed undesirable. On the other hand, if changing the retirement age—particularly the age of early retirement—could induce workers to stay in the labor force longer, this could offset the effect of the reduction in benefits on income and would also provide a greater boost to economic activity than a benefit cut for all retirees. But, those with shorter life expectancies may also have less capacity for work (Cutler, Meara, and Richards-Shubik, 2011). Other possible policies might also face some trade-offs between efficiency and equity. For example, a policy to further means-test benefits might have favorable distributional consequences but would also impose greater implicit taxes on saving.

Tax Increases

Many observers believe that increased tax revenues will be necessary to meet the fiscal challenge posed by population aging. From a macroeconomic standpoint, the particular details of the tax changes are quite important. For example, simply raising tax rates on the existing tax base could have significant disincentive effects on labor force participation as well as on saving, making the required adjustments to the fiscal challenge of aging that much more difficult. On the other hand, many economists believe that reforming the tax code by broadening the base could lead to higher revenues while lowering marginal tax rates. This type of policy could help address the fiscal imbalance while also boosting economic activity.

CONCLUSIONS

A sizable share of the consumption of the elderly is financed by the government, in the form of Social Security, Medicare, and Medicaid. The projected changes in the population's age distribution will create imbalances in these programs and, even under the most optimistic projections, lead to progressively larger budget deficits. The challenges of population aging are made more difficult by rapidly growing health costs and by the underlying structural budget deficits that federal and state and local governments face even in the absence of demographic change. Although government debt can grow faster than the economy for a time, policy changes that increase revenues and/or lower expenditures are inevitable in the next few decades. Analyzing the macroeconomic effects of the potential policy changes requires a consideration of their likely impact on private behavior, which will depend on their timing, their distribution, and their effects on the marginal incentives to work and to invest. To the extent that spending can be reduced and revenues increased in ways that increase economic efficiency, the macroeconomic consequences of the necessary policy changes would be muted.

10

Research Recommendations

In the coming decades the United States will undergo a demographic change as important as any in its history. This change will have significant economic and fiscal effects, many of which have been investigated in the preceding pages. This report confirms what other analyses have posited with regard to the nation's fiscal situation: The fiscal effects of population aging will be very large and will be mediated by how and how quickly our society responds. With regard to macroeconomic effects, the report concludes that while the overall macroeconomic effects of aging may be modest for the economy as a whole, the risks could be large for particular age groups and generations if the burden of adjustment is borne by public programs such as Social Security, Medicare, and Medicaid or if the costs are borne largely by subgroups such as workers or retirees.

Throughout its deliberations, the committee was aware that trends in some of the topics under discussion were, by their nature, speculative. There was a tension between suggesting potential pathways of future change and, at the same time, remaining grounded in empirical knowledge. There were many questions concerning the macroeconomic effects of population aging that the committee thought were important but could not address fully because of a lack of data and/or research. Part of the committee's charge, in response to a request from the Division of Behavioral and Social Research, U.S. National Institute on Aging (NIA), was to identify and recommend major research needs related to the macroeconomics of aging.

This chapter presents the committee's thinking about which additional analyses and lines of inquiry would be most useful, taking into account the feasibility of research on a given topic. Topics have been grouped into four categories: (1) demographic and health measurement and projections; (2) capacity to work and longer working life; (3) changes in consumption and saving; and (4) modeling efforts and data needs. The request from the NIA did not extend to prioritizing a research agenda, and the committee did not attempt to do so. The NIA and other research organizations dealing with questions about an aging society have many competing inputs and priorities, and since the committee did not evaluate them all, the committee felt it was inappropriate to be prescriptive about research priorities. Rather, these recommendations are designed to broadly inform NIA's strategic research direction on the consequences of an aging society and to enable a more complete understanding of the relationship between population aging and the economy in the future.

DEMOGRAPHIC AND HEALTH MEASURES AND PROJECTIONS

1a. Improve methods of projecting mortality by age, sex, and socioeconomic characteristics. Projections of future life expectancy and mortality made by government agencies and demographers differ significantly, in part because projection methods and assumptions differ. The committee believes that increases in life expectancy will likely be more rapid than currently assumed in many projections. Research should consider whether (1) projections could be improved by explicitly taking into account trends in mortality related to smoking, obesity, and other behavioral factors, (2) projections could be improved by taking into account mortality differences by race/ethnicity and educational level (these are particularly important in light of current discussions about increasing the early and full retirement ages, which would have a larger proportional effect on expected years of retired life for groups with lower life expectancy and education), and (3) there is room for further improvement in projections based on formal demographic analysis of past trends and on trends within groups of countries.

1b. Investigate distributional aspects of the relationships between life expectancy, capacity to work, and income. Although the rising disparity in life expectancy across the income distribution has been documented, little is known about the causes of this widening. Similarly, little is known about trends in the capacity to work by income. Understanding the relationship between income distribution, capacity to work, and life expectancy—and having some basis for projecting these trends forward—is important to evaluating the distributional effects of proposals related to raising the eligibility ages for Social Security and Medicare.

1c. Better understand specific risk factors that are precedents of disability, including personal characteristics such as obesity and occupational hazards.

While disability rates among the older U.S. population have been constant over the past decade, disability rates among the working-age population have increased. Rising rates of disability with respect to mobility and related functions, combined with such secular changes as the dramatic increase in overweight and obesity among nonelderly and the tendency for underprivileged populations to drop out of school, suggest that future generations may fare less well than their predecessors. This may affect both the capacity of these future generations to participate in the workforce as they pass through middle age and beyond and also their need for personal care services as they get older.

1d. Quantify the effects of demographic change on state and local government budgets. The fiscal discussion in this report surveyed work to date on the effects of demographic change on state and local government budgets, but much remains to be done. In particular, future research should focus on the impact of demographic change on state and local expenditures for education and health services and on state and local tax revenues, as well as on accurate measurements of the future liabilities for pensions and health benefits for state and local workers (considerable work has been done on the pension side but not on retiree health benefits). Further, an analysis of the potential interactions between federal tax and entitlement policies and state budgets could be important to understanding the total impact of policy reforms: For example, would a delay in the full Social Security or Medicare retirement age have implications for state and local governments?

1e. Evaluate and extend measures and projections of disability/functional status described in this report and elsewhere. U.S. survey data suggest that declines in disability among older persons seen in the 1980s and 1990s have ceased during the past decade. These data generally focus on activities of daily living. Alternative conceptions of functional status sometimes suggest different results. Some researchers are questioning the use of chronological age as a basis for understanding health expectancy and people's views of their own life prospects and have developed alternative measures that address concepts of old-age dependency and work potential. The committee believes the time is ripe for a broad evaluation of different approaches, with an eye to building on work described in this report.

WORK CAPACITY AND INCENTIVES FOR A LONGER WORKING LIFE

**2a. Examine what past relationships between health status, age, and economic incentives for continued work suggest about the likely path of labor force participation rates for older (60-75) workers over the next 30 years. Labor force participation rates have already reversed their long-term decline for men. The average retirement age has risen for women as well, and it appears that the older population is not becoming any less healthy. In view of these and other trends, can we better project labor market activity? There are several elements to this question: (1) What fraction of the older population will have health limitations that prevent them from earning much income at age 62, 65, 68, or even 70? (2) How responsive is labor supply to financial incentives to work? (3) Will the labor market deliver opportunities for older workers that will enable the labor force participation rate to rise significantly? and (4) How might changing labor force patterns among women contribute to the overall labor force participation rate? Part of the research challenge in this area is to distill and synthesize the large quantity of empirical evidence on labor supply response to various factors.

2b. Assess the development and adoption of technologies that enhance the capacity of individuals with specific disabilities to participate in the workforce. There are a number of ways in which policy can affect health and disability in the population. One way in particular would be to encourage the development of technologies, including person-based biomedical advances as well as workplace-based devices, that can help improve the health and capacity of individuals with various types of disabilities to perform job-related functions.

2c. Undertake specific analyses of how work at older ages has been and could be facilitated, including demand-side factors. The analyses within this report strongly suggest that more people will be working to older ages than has been the case in past decades. How long people work will depend not only on health trends and pension incentives, but also on the demand for older workers, opportunities for training, retraining, and continuing education, and the flexibility of work at older ages. As our society moves toward later retirement ages, it will be important to (1) assemble disparate information on the types of arrangements that older workers would prefer; (2) understand the arrangements that firms have created or are willing to think about; and (3) evaluate the effect of any trials.

2d. Study the effects of the health reforms enacted in 2010 (known collectively as the Affordable Care Act, or ACA) on labor force participation. The ACA could have important effects on the retirement decision of older workers and on labor force participation decisions more generally. On the one hand, the ACA will make it easier and less expensive for workers who retire early to purchase health insurance on their own and might thereby encourage more early retirement. On the other hand, it is possible that some potential workers currently remain out of the labor force in order to be eligible for Medicaid or Medicare (through the Social Security disability program). The increased affordability and availability of health insurance under the ACA could raise the labor force participation of these workers. Understanding the magnitude of each of these effects will contribute importantly to our ability to gauge the likely macroeconomic effects of demographic change and to evaluate the likely impacts of various policy reforms.

CHANGES IN CONSUMPTION AND SAVING

3a. Rethink how consumption "needs" change at retirement and how they evolve over the course of the retirement period. One of the most difficult challenges in evaluating the findings on retirement resource adequacy is deciding what the benchmark should be for postretirement consumption. Is an 80 percent replacement rate of income sufficient? Is there a substantial opportunity to substitute home production for market purchases, and do job-related costs represent a substantial share of preretirement consumption spending? How do these factors vary with age and duration of retirements that may last 30 years or more? There have been some studies directed at these issues, but further refinement would contribute to a better understanding of saving adequacy for future cohorts of retirees.

3b. Elucidate the interactions between private saving and government policy. The macroeconomic effects of policy changes depend on how individuals respond to them. In particular, How would households respond to reductions in Social Security or Medicare benefits? A wide empirical literature exists on how the retirement decision is affected by the eligibility age for public pensions, but much less is known about saving behavior and retirement age, or saving behavior and Medicare generosity. Of particular interest, given the likelihood that it will occur, would be the effect on private saving decisions of increased means-testing of benefits.

3c. Evaluate how sensitive retirement preparedness results are to scenarios for financial market returns and changes in health care cost growth. If house prices remain flat in real terms for 10 years, for instance, how would this affect retirement readiness results in 2025? What about a low real return on equities for a decade—a repeat of the 2000-2012 experience, for example? This should be a relatively straightforward set of calculations using extant data from national surveys (e.g., the Health and Retirement Study and the Survey of Consumer Finances) in tandem with projections of asset market movements.

3d. Explore whether and for whom personal saving and labor market attachment will increase with longer lifetimes. If people work longer as their lives are extended, society might be able to pay for old-age income and health care programs targeted at those who cannot self-finance. If people also save more privately, this could reduce their need to draw on public safety-net public programs in old age. But the extent to which various subgroups in the population can and will save more and work longer, as the life cycle lengthens, requires additional research.

MODELING AND DATA

4a. Promote modeling efforts to simulate how demographic aging may interact with changing patterns of health status, labor force participation, saving behavior, and capital market movements. New models of the macroeconomic effects of population aging would allow us to better characterize the sensitivities of projections and the interactions between macroeconomic variables. Resulting simulations would help identify the most important policy levers available now and in the future to influence the adequacy of retirement income. Such analyses can also suggest where coordinated policy actions across several domains can be most productive (e.g., improvements in health and functional status can impact labor force participation and productivity) and reduce the costs of adjustment to demographic aging.

4b. Improve existing models of life-cycle saving and decumulation, and test them with data that link individuals with administrative information on saving, investments, and retirement drawdowns. Longitudinal data collection efforts are critically important for tracking and modeling how older households prepare for, and move into, retirement. Better use of the full range of longitudinal data could provide a real-time means to study policies that influence retirement security. Research also is needed on (1) understanding how improving financial literacy can improve retirement security, including how economic and noneconomic (psychological and sociological) factors interact to affect retirement security, and (2) the effectiveness of financial products and related innovations (e.g., longevity risk pooling, inflation and survivor bonds, and long-term care insurance) that have been and might be developed to help people better manage key risks.

4c. Support and broaden ongoing multidisciplinary survey research. The committee strongly endorses the need for continuing longitudinal surveys that include in a single comprehensive instrument questions on health, functional status, retirement behavior, income, pensions, savings, well-being, planning, and related matters. The Health and Retirement Study (HRS) does exactly this and has been enormously valuable for research on the economics of aging. The availability of comparable longitudinal surveys in many developed and developing nations has greatly enhanced the value of the HRS.

4d. Improve the development and use of macro data. While data at the individual and household level are extremely valuable, it also is useful to have macro-level data on many aspects of economic behavior, disaggregated at least by age and preferably by other variables as well. Data of this sort often can be constructed from existing administrative and survey sources such that no new data collection efforts are needed.

References

Aon Consulting. (2008). *Replacement Ratio Study: A Measurement Tool for Retirement Planning.* Available: http://www.aon.com/about-aon/intellectual-capital/attachments/human-capital-consulting/RRStudy070308.pdf [March 2012].

Apps, P., and Rees, R. (2004). Fertility, taxation and family policy. *Scandinavian Journal of Economics*, 106(4), 745-763.

Arias, E. (2011). United States life tables, 2007. *National Vital Statistics Reports*, 59(9). Hyattsville, MD: National Center for Health Statistics.

Arnott, R.D., and Chaves, D.B. (2011). *Demographic Changes, Financial Markets, and the Economy.* Social Science Research Network Working Paper Series. Available: http://ssrn.com/abstract=1810985 [December 2011].

Attanasio, O., Kitao, S., and Violante, G.L. (2007). Global demographic trends and social security reform. *Journal of Monetary Economics*, 54(1), 144-198.

Auerbach, A.J. (2002). Is there a role for discretionary fiscal policy? In Federal Reserve Board of Kansas City, *Rethinking Stabilization Policy: Proceedings of a Symposium Sponsored by the Federal Reserve Bank of Kansas City* (pp. 109-150). Honolulu: University Press of the Pacific.

Auerbach, A.J. (2003). Fiscal policy, past and present. *Brookings Papers on Economic Activity*, 1, 75-138.

Auerbach, A.J., and Gale, W.G. (2012). *The Federal Budget Outlook: No News Is Bad News.* Tax Policy Center, February 15. Available: http://www.taxpolicycenter.org/UploadedPDF/1001589-The-Budget-Outlook-No-News-Is-Bad-News.pdf [March 2012].

Autor, D.H. (2008). Structural demand shifts and potential labor supply responses in the new century. In K. Bradbury, C.L. Foote, and R.K. Triest (Eds.), *Labor Supply in the New Century* (pp. 161-208). Boston: Federal Reserve Bank of Boston.

Autor, D.H., and Dorn, D. (2011). *The Growth of Low Skill Service Jobs and the Polarization of the U.S. Labor Market.* MIT Working Paper, June. Available: http://econ-www.mit.edu/files/1474 [January 2012].

Autor, D.H., and Duggan, M.G. (2006). The growth in Social Security disability rolls: A fiscal crisis unfolding. *Journal of Economic Perspectives*, 20(3), 71-96.

Avolio, B.J., and Waldman, D.A. (1994). Variations in cognitive, perceptual, and psychomotor abilities across the working life span: Examining the effects of race, sex, experience, education, and occupational type. *Psychology and Aging*, 9(3), 430-442.

Bakshi, G., and Chen, Z. (1994). Baby boom, population aging and capital markets. *Journal of Business*, 67(2), 165-202.

Barro, R.J., Mankiw, N.G., and Sala-i-Martin, X. (1995). Capital mobility in neoclassical models of growth. *American Economic Review*, 85(1), 103-115.

Benzoni, L., Collin-Dufresne, P., and Goldstein, R.S. (2007). Portfolio choice over the life-cycle when the stock and labor markets are cointegrated. *Journal of Finance*, 62(5), 2123-2167.

Bernheim, B.D. (1997). The adequacy of personal retirement saving: Issues and options. In D.A. Wise (Ed.), *Facing the Age Wave* (pp. 30-56). Stanford, CA: Hoover Institution Press.

Bhattacharya, J., Choudhry, K., and Lakdawalla, D. (2008). Chronic disease and severe disability among working-age populations. *Medical Care*, 46, 92-100.

Board of Trustees, Federal Old-Age and Survivors Insurance and Federal Disability Insurance Trust Funds. (2010). *The 2010 Annual Report of the Board of Trustees of the Federal Old-Age and Survivors Insurance and Federal Disability Insurance Trust Funds*. Washington, DC: U.S. Government Printing Office.

Board of Trustees, Federal Old-Age and Survivors Insurance and Federal Disability Insurance Trust Funds. (2011). *The 2011 Annual Report of the Board of Trustees of the Federal Old-Age and Survivors Insurance and Federal Disability Insurance Trust Funds*. Washington, DC: U.S. Government Printing Office.

Board of Trustees, Federal Old-Age and Survivors Insurance and Federal Disability Insurance Trust Funds. (2012). *The 2012 Annual Report of the Board of Trustees of the Federal Old-Age and Survivors Insurance and Federal Disability Insurance Trust Funds*. Washington, DC: U.S. Government Printing Office.

Boards of Trustees, Federal Hospital Insurance and Federal Supplementary Medical Insurance Trust Funds. (2011). *2011 Annual Report of the Boards of Trustees of the Federal Hospital Insurance and Federal Supplemental Medical Insurance Trust Funds*. Washington, DC: U.S. Government Printing Office.

Bodie, Z., Merton, R.C., and Samuelson, W.F. (1992). Labor supply flexibility and portfolio choice in a life cycle model. *Journal of Economic Dynamics and Control*, 16, 427-449.

Boersch-Supan, A., Duezguen, I., and Weiss, M. (2008). Labor productivity in an aging society. In D. Broeders, S. Eijffinger, and A. Houben (Eds.), *Frontiers in Pension Finance and Reform* (pp. 83-96). Cheltenham, U.K.: Edward Elgar.

Boersch-Supan, A.H., and Ludwig, A. (2010). Old Europe is aging: Reforms and reform backlashes. In J.B. Shoven (Ed.), *Demography and the Economy* (pp. 169-204). Chicago: University of Chicago Press.

Boersch-Supan, A., Ludwig, A., and Sommer, M. (2007). *Aging and Asset Prices*. MEA Discussion Paper No. 129-07. Mannheim, Germany: Mannheim Research Institute for the Economics of Aging.

Boersch-Supan, A., Ludwig, A., and Winter, J. (2006). Ageing, pension reform and capital flows: A multi-country simulation model. *Economica*, 73, 625-658.

Boersch-Supan, A.H., Reil-Held, A., and Wilke, C.B. (2007). *How an Unfunded Pension System Looks Like Defined Contributions: The German Pension Reform*. MEA Paper 126-2007. Mannheim, Germany: Mannheim Research Institute for the Economics of Aging. Available: http://mea.mpisoc.mpg.de/uploads/user_mea_discussionpapers/qmdmtjwb7ovclry3_126-07.pdf [February 2012].

Boersch-Supan, A., and Weiss, M. (2011). *Productivity and Age: Evidence from Work Teams at the Assembly Line*. MEA Discussion Paper 148-2007. Mannheim, Germany: Mannheim

Research Institute for the Economics of Aging. Available: http://www.mea.uni-mannheim.de/uploads/user_mea_discussionpapers/1057_MEA-DP_148-2007.pdf [March 2012].

Bongaarts, J. (2006). How long will we live? *Population and Development Review*, 32(4), 605-628.

Brewster, K.L., and Rindfuss, R.R. (2000). Fertility and women's employment in industrialized nations. *Annual Review of Sociology*, 26, 271-296.

Brooks, R. (2002). Asset-market effects of the baby boom and social security reform. *American Economic Review*, 92(2), 402-406.

Brooks, R. (2004). *The Equity Premium and the Baby Boom*. Paper presented at the Econometric Society North American Winter Meetings, San Diego, CA. Available: http://econpapers.repec.org/paper/ecmnawm04/155.htm [November 2011].

Brooks, R. (2006). Demographic change and asset prices. In Reserve Bank of Australia, *RSB Annual Conference Volume* (pp. 236-261). Sydney: Reserve Bank of Australia.

Brown, J., Poterba, J., and Richardson, D.P. (In press). Trends in the distribution decisions of TIAA-CREF participants: 2002-2011. *TIAA-CREF Institute Research Dialogue Issue*.

Bryant, R.C. (2006). *Asymmetric Demographic Transitions and North-South Capital Flows*. Brookings Discussion Papers in International Economics No. 170. Washington, DC: The Brookings Institution.

Bureau of Economic Analysis (BEA). (2011). *A Guide to the National Income and Product Accounts of the United States*. Available: http://www.bea.gov/national/pdf/nipaguid.pdf [January 2012].

Bureau of Labor Statistics (BLS). (2011a). *Download Tables of Multifactor Productivity Measures for Major Sectors and Manufacturing*. Available: http://www.bls.gov/mfp/mprdload.htm [December 2011].

BLS. (2011b). *Labor Force Characteristics of Foreign-Born Workers Summary*. Available: http://www.bls.gov/news.release/forbrn.nr0.htm [September 2011].

BLS. (2012). *Labor Force Statistics from the Current Population Survey*. Available: http://data.bls.gov/pdq/querytool.jsp?survey=ln [March 2012].

Burkhauser, R., and Daly, M. (2011). *The Declining Work and Welfare of People with Disabilities: What Went Wrong and a Strategy for Change*. Washington, DC: American Enterprise Institute Press.

Butrica, B.A., Johnson, R.W., Smith, K.E., and Steurele, E. (2006). The implicit tax on work at older ages. *National Tax Journal*, 59(2), 211-234.

Card, D., and Lemieux, T. (2001). Can falling supply explain the rising return to college for younger men? A cohort-based analysis. *The Quarterly Journal of Economics*, 116(2), 379-420.

Card, D., and Ransom, M. (2011). Pension plan characteristics and framing effects in employee savings behavior. *Review of Economics and Statistics*, 93(1), 228-243.

Carneiro, P., and Lee, S. (2011). Trends in quality-adjusted skill premia in the United States, 1960-2000. *American Economic Review*, 110(6), 2309-2349.

Carnes, B.A., Olshansky, S.J., and Grahn, D. (1996). Continuing the search for a law of mortality. *Population and Development Review*, 22(2), 231-264.

Carnevale, A., Smith, N., and Strohl, J. (2010). *Help Wanted: Projections of Jobs and Education Requirements Through 2018*. Washington, DC: Georgetown University Center on Education and the Workforce.

Centers for Disease Control and Prevention. (2011). CDC health disparities and inequalities report—United States, 2011. *Morbidity and Mortality Weekly Report*, 60 (Supplement). Available: http://www.cdc.gov/mmwr/pdf/other/su6001.pdf [January 2011].

Centers for Medicare and Medicaid Services. (2011a). *Data Compendium. 2010 Edition*. Available: https://www.cms.gov/DataCompendium/14_2010_Data_Compendium.asp [February 2012].

Centers for Medicare and Medicaid Services. (2011b). *Health Expenditures by Age*. Available: https://www.cms.gov/NationalHealthExpendData/downloads/2004-age-tables.pdf [February 2012].

Chai, J., Horneff, W., Maurer, R., and Mitchell, O.S. (2011). Optimal portfolio choice over the life cycle with flexible work, endogenous retirement, and lifetime payouts. *Review of Finance*, 15(4), 875-907.

Chen, Y.-P., and Scott, J.C. (2006). Phased retirement: Who opts for it and toward what end? *European Papers on the New Welfare*, 6, 16-28.

Choi, J., Laibson, D., Madrian, B., and Metrick, A. (2002). Defined contribution pensions: Plan rules, participant decisions, and the path of least resistance. In J.M. Poterba (Ed.), *Tax Policy and the Economy, Volume 16* (pp. 67-114). Chicago: University of Chicago Press.

Christensen, K., and Vaupel, J.W. (2011). Genetic factors and adult mortality. In R.G. Rogers and E.M. Crimmins (Eds.), *International Handbook of Adult Mortality* (pp. 399-410). New York: Springer.

Congressional Budget Office (CBO). (2008) Growing disparities in life expectancy. *Economic and Budget Issue Brief*, April 17. Available: http://www.cbo.gov/ftpdocs/91xx/doc9104/04-17-LifeExpectancy_Brief.pdf [January 2012].

CBO. (2011). *CBO's 2011 Long-Term Budget Outlook*. Publication No. 4277. Washington, DC: Congressional Budget Office.

CBO. (2012). *Updated Budget Projections: Fiscal Years 2012 to 2022*. Available: http://www.cbo.gov/sites/default/files/cbofiles/attachments/March 2012Baseline.pdf [March 2012].

Copeland, C. (2011). Labor-force participation rates of the population age 55 and older: What did the recession do to the trends? *Employee Benefit Research Institute Notes*, 32(2), 8-16.

Coronado, J., and Dynan, K. (In press). Changing retirement behavior in the wake of the financial crisis. In O.S. Mitchell, R. Maurer and M. Warshawsky (Eds.), *Reshaping Retirement Security: Lessons from the Global Financial Crisis*. Oxford, U.K.: Oxford University Press.

Costa, D.L. (1998). *The Evolution of Retirement: An American Economic History, 1880-1990*. Chicago: University of Chicago Press.

Crimmins, E.M., and Beltrán-Sánchez, H. (2011). Mortality and morbidity trends: Is there compression of morbidity? *The Journals of Gerontology, Series B*, 66(1), 75-86.

Crimmins, E.M., Kim, J.K., and Seeman, T.E. (2009). Poverty and biological risk: The earlier "aging" of the poor. *The Journals of Gerontology, Series A*, 64(2), 286-292.

Cutler, D.M., and Lleras-Muney, A. (2006). *Education and Health: Evaluating Theories and Evidence*. NBER Working Paper No. 12352. Cambridge, MA: National Bureau of Economic Research.

Cutler, D.M., and Lleras-Muney, A. (2010). Understanding differences in health behaviors by education. *Journal of Health Economics*, 29, 1-28.

Cutler, D.M., Meara, E., and Richards-Shubik, S. (2011). *Healthy Life Expectancy: Estimates and Implications for Retirement Age Policy*. NBER Working Paper No. NB10-11. Cambridge, MA: National Bureau of Economic Research.

Cutler, D.M., Poterba, J.M., Sheiner, L.M., and Summers, L.H. (1990). An aging society: Opportunity or challenge?" *Brookings Papers on Economic Activity*, 21(1), 1-73.

Cutler, D.M., and Sheiner, L. (2001). Demographics and medical care spending: Standard and non-standard effects. In A.J. Auerbach and R.D. Lee (Eds.), *Demographic Change and Fiscal Policy* (pp. 253-291). Cambridge, U.K.: Cambridge University Press.

Department of Labor. (2010). *Quick Stats on Women Workers, 2010*. Available: http://www.dol.gov/wb/factsheets/QS-womenwork2010.htm [December 2011].

DiCecio, R., Engemann, K.M., Owyang, M.T., and Wheeler, C.H. (2008). Changing trends in the labor force: A survey. *Federal Reserve Bank of St. Louis Review*, 90(1), 47-62.

Donehower, G., and Boe, C. (2012). *Population and Related Projections Made by the Committee*. Appendix prepared for the report of the National Research Council Committee on the Long-Run Macroeconomic Effects of the Aging U.S. Population.

Elinson, L., Houck, P., Marcus, S.C., and Pincus, H.A. (2004). Depression and the ability to work. *Psychiatric Services*, 55(1), 29-34.

Elo, I.T., and Preston, S.H. (1997). Racial and ethnic differences in mortality at older ages. In L.G. Martin and B.J. Soldo (Eds.), *Racial and Ethnic Differences in the Health of Older Americans* (pp. 10-42). National Research Council. Washington, DC: National Academy Press.

Employee Benefit Research Institute (EBRI). (2009). *Savings Needed for Health Expenses in Retirement: An Examination of Persons Aged 55 and 65 in 2009*. EBRI Notes, 30(6). Washington, DC: Employee Benefit Research Institute.

EBRI. (2011a). *Employment-Based Retirement Plan Participation: Geographic Differences and Trends, 2010*. EBRI Issue Brief 363. Washington, DC: Employee Benefit Research Institute.

EBRI. (2011b). Workers' Pessimism About Retirement Deepens, Reflecting "the New Normal." Press Release. Available: http://www.ebri.org/pdf/surveys/rcs/2011/PR914_15Mar11_RCS.pdf [March 2012].

Engelhardt, H., and Prskawetz, A. (2004). On the changing correlation between fertility and female employment over space and time. *European Journal of Population*, 20, 35-62.

Ezzati, M., Friedman, A.B., Kulkarni, S.C., and Murray, C.J.L. (2008). The reversal of fortunes: Trends in county mortality and cross-county mortality disparities in the United States. *PLoS Medicine*, 5(4), 557-568.

Federal Reserve. (2011). *Flow of Funds Accounts of the United States*. Statistical Release. Available: http://www.federalreserve.gov/releases/z1/ [August 2011].

Federal Reserve Board of San Francisco. (2005). Housing markets and demographics. *FRBSF Economic Letter*, 2005-21 (August 26). Available: http://www.frbsf.org/publications/economics/letter/2005/el2005-21.pdf [June 2012].

Feyrer, J. (2007). Demographics and productivity. *Review of Economics and Statistics*, 89(1), 100-109.

Feyrer, J. (2008). Aggregate evidence on the link between age structure and productivity. *Population and Development Review*, 34, 78-99.

Freedman, V.A. (2011). Disability, functioning and aging. In R.H. Binstock and L.K. George, (Eds.), *Handbook of Aging and the Social Sciences*. Seventh Edition (pp. 57-73). San Diego: Academic Press.

Freedman, V.A., Agree, E.M., Martin, L.G., and Cornman, J. (2006). Trends in the use of assistive technology and personal care for late-life disability, 1992-2001. *The Gerontologist*, 46, 124-127.

Freedman, V.A., Crimmins, E.M., Schoeni, R.F., Spillman, B., Aykan, H., Kramarow, E., Land, K., Manton, K., Martin, L.G., Shinberg, D., and Waidmann, T. (2004). Resolving inconsistencies in old-age disability trends: Report from a technical working group. *Demography*, 41(3), 417-441.

Freedman, V.A., Kaspar, J.D., Cornman, J.C., Agree, E.M., Bandeen-Roche, K., Mor, V., Spillman, B.C., Wallace, R., and Wolf, D.A. (2011). Validation of new measures of disability and functioning in the national health and aging trends study. *The Journals of Gerontology, Series A*, 66(9), 1013-1021.

Freedman, V.A., Spillman, B., Andreski, P., Cornman, J.C., Crimmins, E., Kramarow, E., Lubitz, J., Martin, L., Merkin, S., Schoeni, R.F., Seeman, T., and Waidmann, T. (In press). Trends in late-life activity limitations: An update from 5 national surveys. *Demography*.

Fries, J.F. (1980). Aging, natural death, and the compression of morbidity. *New England Journal of Medicine*, 303, 1369-1370.
Furtado, D., and Hock, H. (2008). *Immigrant Labor, Child-Care Services, and the Work-Fertility Trade-Off in the United States*. IZA Discussion Papers (May). Available: http://ideas.repec.org/p/iza/izadps/dp3506.html [August 2011].
Furtado, D., and Hock, H. (2010). Low skilled immigration and work-fertility tradeoffs among high skilled US natives. *American Economic Review*, 100(2), 224-228.
Galenson, D.W. (2004a). *A Portrait of the Artist as a Young or Old Innovator: Measuring the Careers of Modern Novelists*. NBER Working Paper No. 10213. Cambridge, MA: National Bureau of Economic Research.
Galenson, D.W. (2004b). *A Portrait of the Artist as a Very Young or Very Old Innovator: Creativity at the Extremes of the Lifecycle*. NBER Working Paper No. 10515. Cambridge, MA: National Bureau of Economic Research.
Galor, O., and Weil, D.N. (1996). The gender gap, fertility, and growth. *American Economic Review*, 86(3), 374-387.
Geanakoplos, J., Magill, M., and Quinzii, M. (2004). Demography and the long-run predictability of the stock market. *Brookings Papers on Economic Activity*, 1, 241-307.
Gendell, M. (2008). Older workers: Increasing their labor force participation and hours of work. *Monthly Labor Review*, January, 41-54.
Goda, G.S., Shoven, J.B., and Slavov, S.N. (2007). *A Tax on Work for the Elderly: Medicare as a Secondary Payer*. NBER Working Paper No. 13383. Cambridge, MA: National Bureau of Economic Research.
Goda, G.S., Shoven, J.B., and Slavov, S.N. (2009). Removing the disincentive in social security for long careers. In J. Brown, J. Liebman, and D.A. Wise (Eds). *Social Security Policy in a Changing Environment*. Chicago: University of Chicago Press.
Goda, G.S., Shoven, J.B., and Slavov, S.N. (2011). Implicit taxes on work from Social Security and Medicare. In J. Brown (Ed.), *Tax Policy and the Economy (Volume 25)*. Chicago: University of Chicago Press.
Government Accountability Office (GAO). (2010). *Social Security Reform. Raising the Retirement Ages Would Have Implications for Older Workers and SSA Disability Rolls*. GAO-11-125. Available: http://www.gao.gov/new.items/d11125.pdf [December 2011].
GAO. (2012). *State and Local Governments' Fiscal Outlook. April 2012 update*. GAO-12-523SP. Available: http://www.gao.gov/products/GAO-12-523SP [April 2012].
Green, R.K., and Hendershott, P.H. (1996). Age, demographics and real house prices. *Regional Science and Urban Economics*, 26(5), 465-480.
Greenwald, M., Kapteyn, A., Mitchell, O.S., and Schneider, L. (2010). *What Do People Know About Social Security?* RAND Financial Literacy Center. Available: http://www.rand.org/labor/centers/financial-literacy/projects/social-security-benefits.html [December 2011].
Griliches, Z. (1990). Patent statistics as economic indicators. *Journal of Economic Literature*, 28(4), 1661-1707.
Gruber, J. (2009). *Public Finance and Public Policy*. New York: Worth Publishers.
Gruber, J., and Wise, D.A. (1999). Introduction and summary. In J. Gruber and D.A. Wise (Eds.), *Social Security and Retirement Around the World* (pp. 1-35). Chicago: University of Chicago Press.
Gruber, J., and Wise, D.A. (2007). Introduction and summary. In J. Gruber and D.A. Wise (Eds.), *Social Security Programs and Retirement Around the World: Fiscal Implications* (pp. 1-42). Chicago: University of Chicago Press.
Gruber, J., Milligan, K.S., and Wise, D.A. (2009). Introduction and summary. In J. Gruber and D.A. Wise (Eds.), *Social Security Programs and Retirement Programs Around the World: The Relationship to Youth Employment* (pp. 1-45). Chicago: University of Chicago Press.

Guidolin, M., and La Jeunesse, E.A. (2007). The decline in the U.S. personal savings rate: Is it real and is it a puzzle? *Federal Reserve Bank of St. Louis Review*, 89(6), 491-514.

Gustman, A.L., and Steinmeier, T.L. (2002). *The Social Security Entitlement Age in a Structural Model of Retirement and Wealth*. NBER Working Paper No. 9183. Cambridge, MA: National Bureau of Economic Research.

Gustman, A.L., Steinmeier, T.L., and Tabatabai, N. (2010). *Pensions in the Health and Retirement Study*. Cambridge, MA: Harvard University Press.

Haber, C., and Gratton, B. (1994). *Old Age and the Search for Security*. Bloomington: Indiana University Press.

Hamilton, B.W. (1991). The baby boom, the baby bust, and the housing market. A second look. *Regional Science and Urban Economics*, 21(4), 547-552.

Hammond, P.B., and Richardson, D.P. (2009). Staying on the path to a secure retirement: Using the asset-salary ratio as a retirement compass. *TIAA-CREF Institute Research Dialogue Issue 95*. Available: http://www.tiaa-cref.org/ institute/research/dialogue/rd_assetsalaryratio1209.html [December 2011].

Hanna, S.D., and Lindamood, S. (2004). An improved measure of risk aversion. *Financial Counseling and Planning*, 15(2), 27-38.

Hariharana, G., Chapman, K.G., and Domian, D.L. (2000). Risk tolerance and asset allocation for investors nearing retirement. *Financial Services Review*, 9, 159-170.

Haveman, R., and Wolfe, B. (2000). The economics of disability and disability policy. In A.J. Cutler and J.P. Newhouse (Eds.), *Handbook of Health Economics* (pp. 996-1051). Chicago: Elsevier Science.

Haveman, R., Holden, K., Wolfe, B.L., and Romanov, A. (2007). The sufficiency of retirement savings: Comparing cohorts at the time of retirement. In B. Madrian, O.S. Mitchell, and B.J. Soldo (Eds.), *Redefining Retirement: How Will Boomers Fare?* (pp. 36-69). New York: Oxford University Press.

He, W., Sengupta, M., Velkoff, V.A., and DeBarros, K.A. (2005). *65+ in the United States: 2005*, U.S. Census Bureau Current Population Report P23-209. Washington, DC: U.S. Government Printing Office.

Health and Retirement Study. University of Michigan. See: http://hrsonline.isr.umich.edu/

Hoorens, S., Clift, J., Staetsky, L., Janta, B., Diepeveen, S., Morgan Jones, M., and Grant, J. (2011). *Low Fertility in Europe*. RAND Europe. Available: http://www.rand.org/content/dam/rand/pubs/monographs/2011/RAND_MG1080.pdf [December 2011].

Hummer, R.A., and Lariscy, J.T. (2011). Educational attainment and adult mortality. In R.G. Rogers and E.M. Crimmins (Eds.), *International Handbook of Adult Mortality* (pp. 241-262). New York: Springer.

Hurd, M.D., and McGarry, K. (1995). Evaluation of the subjective probabilities of survival in the Health and Retirement Study. *Journal of Human Resources*, 30(Special Issue), S268-S292.

International Monetary Fund. (2011). *World Economic Outlook*. Washington, DC: International Monetary Fund.

Issa, P., and Zedlewski, S.R. (2011). *Poverty Among Older Americans, 2009*. Urban Institute Retirement Security Brief. Available: http://www.urban.org/uploadedpdf/412296-Poverty-Among-Older-Americans.pdf [March 2012].

Iwry, J.M. (2004). Testimony before the Committee on Education and the Workforce, Subcommittee on Employer-Employee Relations, U.S. House of Representatives, April 29. Available: http://archives.republicans.edlabor.house.gov/archive/hearings/108th/eer/pensions04 2904/iwry.htm [December 2011].

Jagannathan, R., and Kocherlakota, N.R. (1996). Why should older people invest less in stocks than younger people? *Federal Reserve Bank of Minneapolis Quarterly Review*, 20(3), 11-23.

James, B.D., Boyle, P.A., Buchman, A.S., and Bennett, D.A. (2011). Relation of late-life social activity with incident disability among community-dwelling older adults. *The Journals of Gerontology, Biological and Medical Sciences*, 66A(4), 467-473.
Johnson, R., Toohey, D., and Wiener, J.M. (2007). *Meeting the Long-Term Care Needs of the Baby Boomers: How Changing Families Will Affect Paid Helpers and Institutions.* Urban Institute Discussion Paper 04-07. Washington, DC: Urban Institute.
Jones, B.F. (2009). The burden of knowledge and the death of the Renaissance man: Is innovation getting harder? *Review of Economic Studies*, 76(1), 283-317.
Jones, B.F. (2010). Age and great invention. *Review of Economics and Statistics*, 92(1), 1-14.
Jones, C.I., and Romer, P.M. (2010). The new Kaldor facts: Ideas, institutions, population, and human capital. *American Economic Journal: Macroeconomics*, 2(1), 224-245.
Juhn, C., and Potter, S. (2006). Changes in labor force participation in the United States. *Journal of Economic Perspectives*, 20(3), 27-46.
Kapteyn, A., and Teppa, F. (2011). Subjective measures of risk aversion, fixed costs, and portfolio choice. *Journal of Economic Psychology*, 32(4), 564-580.
Karoly, L.A., and Panis, C.W.A. (2004). *The 21st Century at Work*. Santa Monica, CA: RAND Corporation.
Kawachi, I., Adler, N.E., and Dow, W.H. (2010). Money, schooling, and health: Mechanisms and causal evidence. *Annals of the New York Academy of Sciences*, 1186, 56-68.
Kohler, H.-P., Billari, F.C., and Ortega, J.A. (2006). Low fertility in Europe: Causes, implications and policy options. In F.R. Harris (Ed.), *The Baby Bust: Who Will Do the Work? Who Will Pay the Taxes?* (pp. 48-109). Lanham, MD: Rowman & Littlefield.
Kotlikoff, L.J., and Wise, D.A. (1988). Pension backloading, implicit wage taxes, and work disincentives. In L.H. D Summers (Ed.), *Tax Policy and the Economy: Volume 2* (pp. 161-196). Boston: MIT Press.
Kotlikoff, L.J., and Wise, D.A. (1989). Employee retirement and a firm's pension plan. In D.A. Wise (Ed.), *The Economics of Aging* (pp. 279-334). Chicago: University of Chicago Press.
Krüger, D., and Ludwig, A. (2007). On the consequences of demographic change for rates of returns to capital, and the distribution of wealth and welfare. *Journal of Monetary Economics*, 54(1), 49-87.
Kuhle, W. (2008). *Demography and Equity Premium*. MEA Discussion Paper No. 157-08. Mannheim, Germany: Mannheim Research Institute for the Economics of Aging.
Lacey, T.A., and Wright, B. (2009). Occupational employment projections to 2018. *Monthly Labor Review*, November, 82-123.
Lee, M.A., and Mather, M. (2008). U.S. labor force trends. *Population Bulletin*, No. 63. Washington, DC: Population Reference Bureau.
Lee, R.D. (1999). Probabilistic approaches to population forecasting. *Population and Development Review*, 24(Supplement), 156-190.
Lee, R.D. (2011). The outlook for population growth. *Science*, 333, 569-573.
Lee, R.D., and Carter, L.R. (1992). Modeling and forecasting U.S. mortality. *Journal of the American Statistical Association*, 87(419), 659-671.
Lee, R.D., Donehower, G., and Miller, T. (2011). The changing shape of the economic lifecycle in the United States, 1960 to 2003. In R.D. Lee and A. Mason (Eds.), *Population Aging and the Generational Economy. A Global Perspective* (pp. 313-326). Cheltenham, U.K.: Edward Elgar.
Lee, R.D., and Mason, A. (Eds). (2011). *Population Aging and the Generational Economy. A Global Perspective*. Cheltenham, U.K.: Edward Elgar.
Lee, R.D., and Miller, T. (2002). An approach to forecasting health expenditures with application to the U.S. Medicare system. *Health Services Research*, 3(5), 1365-1386.

REFERENCES

Lee, R.D., and Tuljapurkar, S. (1994). Stochastic population projections for the United States: Beyond high, medium and low. *Journal of the American Statistical Association*, 89(428), 1175-1189.

Lehman, H.C. (1953). *Age and Achievement*. Princeton, NJ: Princeton University Press.

Lemieux, T. (2006). The 'Mincer equation' thirty years after schooling, experience, and earnings. In S. Grossbard (Ed.), *Jacob Mincer. A Pioneer of Modern Labor Economics* (Part IV, pp.127-145). London, U.K.: Springer Verlag.

Levine, P.B., and Mitchell, O.S. (1988). The baby boom's legacy: Relative wages in the twenty-first century. *American Economic Review*, 78(2), 66-69.

Levy, F. (2010). *How Technology Changes Demands for Human Skills*. OECD Education Working Paper No. 45. Paris: Organisation for Economic Co-operation and Development.

Li, N., and Lee, R.D. (2005). Coherent mortality forecasts for a group of populations: An extension of the Lee-Carter method. *Demography*, 42(3), 575-594.

Liu, Z., and Spiegel, M.M. (2011). Boomer retirement: Headwinds for U.S. equity markets? *Federal Reserve Bank of San Francisco Economic Letter*, 2011(26). Available:http://www.frbsf.org/publications/economics/letter/2011/el2011-26.html [December 2011].

Ludwig, A., Krüger, D., and Boersch-Supan, A. (2007). *Demographic Change, Relative Factor Prices, International Capital Flows, and Their Differential Effects on the Welfare of Generations*. NBER Working Paper No. 13185. Cambridge, MA: National Bureau of Economic Research.

Ludwig, A., Schelkle, T., and Vogel, E. (2010). *Demographic Change, Human Capital and Welfare*. MEA Discussion Paper No. 196-10. Mannheim, Germany: Mannheim Research Institute for the Economics of Aging.

Lumsdaine, R.L., Stock, J.H., and Wise, D.A. (1997). Retirement incentives: The interaction between employer-provided pensions, Social Security, and retiree health benefits. In M.D. Hurd and N. Yashiro (Eds.), *The Economic Effects of Aging in the United States and Japan* (261-293). Chicago: University of Chicago Press.

Lusardi, A., and Mitchell, O.S. (2007a). Baby boomer retirement security: The roles of planning, financial literacy, and housing wealth. *Journal of Monetary Economics*, 54, 205-224.

Lusardi, A., and Mitchell, O.S. (2007b). *Financial Literacy and Retirement Planning: New Evidence from the Rand American Life Panel*. Michigan Retirement Research Center Working Paper No. 2007-157. Ann Arbor: Michigan Retirement Research Center.

Lusardi, A., and Mitchell, O.S. (2007c). Financial literacy and retirement preparedness: Evidence and implications for financial education. *Business Economics*, 42(1), 35-44.

Lusardi, A., and Mitchell, O.S. (2009). Financial literacy: Evidence and implications for financial education. *TIAA-CREF Institute Trends and Issues*, May. Available: http://www.tiaa crefinstitute.org/institute/research/trends_issues/ti_financialliter acv0509.html [December 2011].

Lusardi, A., and Mitchell, O.S. (2011). *Financial Literacy Around the World: An Overview*. Netspar Discussion Paper 02/2011-023. Available: http://papers.ssrn.com/sol3/papers.cfm?abstract_id=1810551 [February 2012].

Lusardi, A., Mitchell, O.S., and Curto, V. (2010). Financial literacy among the young: Evidence and implications for consumer policy. *Journal of Consumer Affairs*, 44(2), 358-380.

Lutz, W., Sanderson, W.C., and Scherbov, S. (Eds). (2004). *The End of World Population Growth in the 21st Century. New Challenges for Human Capital Formation and Sustainable Development*. London: Earthscan.

Lybbert, T.J., and Just, D.R. (2007). Is risk aversion really correlated with wealth? How estimated probabilities introduce spurious correlation. *American Journal of Agricultural Economics*, 89(4), 964-979.

MacArthur Foundation Research Network on an Aging Society. (2009). Facts and fictions about an aging America. *Contexts*, 8(4), 16-21.

Mankiw, N.G., and Weil, D. (1989). The baby boom, the baby bust, and the housing market. *Regional Science and Urban Economics*, 19, 235-258.

Manyika, J., Lund, S., Auguste, B., Mendonca, L., Welsh, T., and Ramaswamy, S. (2011). *An Economy That Works: Job Creation and America's Future*. Washington, DC: McKinsey Global Institute.

Markides, K.S., and Eschbach, K. (2011). Hispanic paradox in adult mortality in the United States. In R.G. Rogers and E.M. Crimmins (Eds.), *International Handbook of Adult Mortality* (pp. 227-240). New York: Springer.

Martin, L.G., Freedman, V.A., Schoeni, R.F., and Andreski, P.M. (2009). Health and functioning among baby boomers approaching 60. *The Journals of Gerontology, Psychological Sciences and Social Sciences*, 64B(3), 369-377.

Martin, L.G., Schoeni, R.F., and Andreski, P.M. (2010). Trends in health of older adults in the United States: Past, present, future. *Demography*, 47(Supplement), S17-S40.

Martínez, D.F., and Iza, A. (2004). Skill premium effects on fertility and female labor force supply. *Journal of Population Economics*, 17(1), 1-16.

Mason, A., and Lee, R.D. (2011). Introducing age into national accounts. In R.D. Lee and A. Mason (Eds.), *Population Aging and the Generational Economy. A Global Perspective* (pp. 55-78). Cheltenham, U.K.: Edward Elgar.

McFadden, D. (1994). Demographics, the housing market, and the welfare of the elderly. In D.A. Wise (Ed.), *Studies in the Economics of Aging* (pp. 225-88). Chicago: University of Chicago Press.

McGill, D., Brown, K.N., Haley, J.J., Schieber, S., and Warshawsky, M.J. (2010). *Fundamentals of Private Pensions*. Oxford, U.K.: Oxford University Press.

McKinsey Global Institute. (2009). *Changing the Fortunes of America's Workforce: A Human Capital Challenge*. Washington, DC: McKinsey and Company.

Milligan, K.S., and Wise, D.A. (2011). *Social Security and Retirement Around the World: Historical Trends in Mortality and Health, Employment, and Disability Insurance Participation and Reforms—Introduction and Summary*. NBER Working Paper No. 16719. Cambridge, MA: National Bureau of Economic Research.

Mitchell, O.S., and Lusardi, A. (Eds.). (2011). *Financial Literacy: Implications for Retirement Security and the Financial Marketplace*. Oxford: Oxford University Press.

Mitchell, O.S., and Moore, J. (1997). *Retirement Wealth Accumulation and Decumulation: New Developments and Outstanding Opportunities*. Wharton Financial Institutions Center Working Paper 97-12. Available: http://fic.wharton.upenn.edu/fic/papers/97/9712.pdf.

Mitchell, O.S., and Moore, J. (1998). Can Americans afford to retire? New evidence on retirement saving adequacy. *Journal of Risk and Insurance*, 65(3), 371-400.

Mitchell, O.S., Piggott, J., Sherris, M., and Yow, S. (2006). Financial innovations for an aging world. In C. Kent, A. Park, and D. Rees (Eds.), *Demography and Financial Markets* (pp. 299-336). Sydney: Pegasus Press.

Mitchell, O.S., Piggott, J., and Takayama, N. (Eds.). (2011). *Revisiting Retirement Payouts: Market Developments and Policy Issues*. New York: Oxford University Press.

Molla, M.T., Madans, J.H., and Wagener, D.K. (2004). Differentials in adult mortality and activity limitation by years of education in the United States at the end of the 1990s. *Population and Development Review*, 30(4), 625-664.

Moon, M., and Smeeding, T.M. (1980). Valuing government expenditures: The case of medical care transfers and poverty. *Review of Income and Wealth*, 26(3), 305-323.

Morin, R.A., and Suarez, A.F. (1983). Risk aversion revisited. *The Journal of Finance*, 38(4), 1201-1216.

Munnell, A., Aubry, J.-P., Hurwitz, J., and Quinby, L. (2011). Can state and local pensions muddle through? *State and Local Pension Plans*, 15. Boston College Center for Retirement Research. Available: http://crr.bc.edu/images/stories/Briefs/slp_15.pdf [February 2012].

Munnell, A.H., and Soto, M. (2005). *What Replacement Rates Do Households Actually Experience in Retirement?* Center for Retirement Research Working Paper No. 2005-10. Chestnut Hill, MA: Center for Retirement Research at Boston College.

Murphy, K.M., and Welch, F. (1990). Empirical age-earnings profiles. *Journal of Labor Economics*, 8, 202-229.

Nagi, S.Z. (1965). Some conceptual issues in disability and rehabilitation. In M.B. Sussman (Ed.), *Sociology and Rehabilitation* (pp. 100-113). Washington, DC: American Sociological Association.

National Bureau of Economic Research. International Social Security Project. Available: http://www.nber.org/booksbyseries/ISS.html.

National Center for Health Statistics. (2011). Births: Preliminary data for 2010. *National Vital Statistics Report*, 60(2). Available: http://www.cdc.gov/nchs/data/nvsr/nvsr60/nvsr60 _02.pdf [March 2012].

National Institute on Aging. (2007). *Growing Older in America. The Health & Retirement Study*. Bethesda, MD: National Institute on Aging.

National Research Council (NRC). (1990). *On Time to the Doctorate: A Study of the Lengthening Time to Completion for Doctorates in Science and Engineering*. H. Tuckman, S. Coyle, and Y. Bae (Eds.). Washington, DC: National Academy Press.

NRC. (1997). *The New Americans. Economic, Demographic, and Fiscal Effects of Immigration*. J.P. Smith and B. Edmonston (Eds.). Washington, DC: National Academy Press.

NRC. (1998). *Trends in the Early Careers of Life Scientists*. Washington, DC: National Academy Press.

NRC. (2000). *Beyond Six Billion: Forecasting the World's Population*. J. Bongaarts and R.A. Bulatao (Eds). Washington, DC: National Academy Press.

NRC. (2001). *America Becoming: Racial Trends and Their Consequences*. N.J. Smelser, W.J. Wilson, and F. Mitchell (Eds.). Washington, DC: National Academy Press.

NRC. (2004a). *Critical Perspectives on Racial and Ethnic Differences in Health in Late Life*. N.B. Anderson, R.A. Bulatao, and B. Cohen (Eds.). Washington, DC: The National Academies Press.

NRC. (2004b). *Understanding Racial and Ethnic Differences in Health in Late Life: A Research Agenda*. R.A. Bulatao and N.B. Anderson (Eds.). Washington, DC: The National Academies Press.

NRC. (2011). *Explaining Divergent Levels of Longevity in High Income Countries*. E.M. Crimmins, S.H. Preston, and B. Cohen (Eds.) Washington, DC: The National Academies Press.

NRC and National Academy of Public Administration. (2010). *Choosing the Nation's Fiscal Future*. Washington, DC: The National Academies Press.

Novy-Marx, R., and Rauh, J. (2010). Public pension promises: How big are they and what are they worth? *Journal of Finance*, 66(4), 1211-1249.

Nyce, S., Schieber, S., Shoven, J.B., Slavov, S., and Wise, D.A. (2011). *Does Retiree Health Insurance Encourage Early Retirement?* NBER Working Paper No. 17703. Cambridge, MA: National Bureau of Economic Research.

O'Brien, E. (2005). *Long-Term Care: Understanding Medicaid's Role for the Elderly and Disabled*. Report prepared for the Kaiser Commission on Medicaid and the Uninsured. Available: http://www.kff.org/medicaid/upload/Long-Term-Care-Understanding-Medicaid-s-Role-for-the-Elderly-and-Disabled-Report.pdf [January 2012].

Oeppen, J., and Vaupel, J.W. (2002). Broken limits to life expectancy. *Science*, 296, 1029-1031.

Ogden, C.L., Carroll, M.D., Curtin, L.R., McDowell, M.A., Tabak, C.J., and Flegal, K.M. (2006). Prevalence of overweight and obesity in the United States, 1999-2004. *Journal of the American Medical Association*, 295, 1549-1552.

Ogden, C.L., Yanovski, F.Z., Carroll, M.D., and Flegal, K.M. (2007). The epidemiology of obesity. *Gastroenterology*, 132, 2087-2102.

Olshansky, S.J., Antonucci, T., Berkman, L., Binstock, R.H., Boersch-Supan, Axel, Cacioppo, J.T., Carnes, B.A., Carstensen, L.L., Fried, L.P., Goldman, D.P., Jackson, J., Kohli, M., Rother, J., Zheng, Y., and Rowe, J. (2012). Differences in life expectancy due to race and educational differences are widening, and many may not catch up. *Health Affairs*, 31(8), 1-11.

Olshansky, S.J., Passaro, D.J., Hershow, R.C., Layden, J., Carnes, B.A., Brody, J., Hayflick, L., Butler, R.N., Allison, D.B., and Ludwig, D.S. (2005). A potential decline in life expectancy in the United States in the 21st century. *New England Journal of Medicine*, 352, 1138-1145.

Organisation for Economic Co-operation and Development (OECD). (2009). *Life-Expectancy Links. The Quiet Revolution in Pension Policy.* Available: http://www.oecd.org/data oecd/41/24/39468250.pdf [January 2012].

OECD. (2010). *Average Effective Age at Retirement.* Available: http://www.oecd.org/data oecd/3/1/39371913.xls [July 2011].

OECD. (2011). *OECD Health Data 2011.* Available: http://stats.oecd.org/index.aspx? DataSetCode=HEALTH_STAT [October 2011].

Paravisini, D., Rappoport, V., and Ravine, E. (2010). *Risk Aversion and Wealth: Evidence from Person-to-Person Lending Portfolios.* NBER Working Paper 16063. Cambridge, MA: National Bureau of Economic Research.

Parrado, E.A. (2011). How high is Hispanic/Mexican fertility in the United States? Immigration and tempo considerations. *Demography*, 48(3), 1059-1080.

Pension Benefit Guarantee Corporation. (2011). *2011 PBGC Annual Report.* Available: http://www.pbgc.gov/res/reports/ar2011.html [May 2012].

Perun, P., and Steuerle, C.E. (2006). Reality testing for pension reform. In R.L. Clark and O.S. Mitchell (Eds.), *Reinventing the Retirement Paradigm* (pp. 36-51). Oxford, U.K.: Oxford University Press.

Poterba, J. (2001). Demographic structure and asset returns. *Review of Economics and Statistics*, 83(4), 565-584.

Poterba, J., Venti, S., and Wise, D.A. (2010). *The Asset Cost of Poor Health.* NBER Working Paper No. 16389. Cambridge, MA: National Bureau of Economic Research.

Poterba, J., Venti, S., and Wise, D.A. (2011). The composition and draw-down of wealth in retirement. *Journal of Economic Perspectives*, 25(4), 95-118.

Prskawetz, A., and Lindh, T. (Eds.). (2006). *The Impact of Population Ageing on Innovation and Productivity Growth in Europe.* Austrian Academy of Sciences Research Report 28. Vienna: Austrian Academy of Sciences.

Psacharopoulos, G., and Patrinos, H.A. (2002). *Returns to Investment in Education: A Further Update.* Policy Research Working Paper Series No. 2881. Washington, DC: The World Bank.

Purcell, P. (2007). *Older Workers: Employment and Retirement Trends.* Congressional Research Service. Available: http://digitalcommons.ilr.cornell.edu/key_ workplace/308/ [May 2010].

Purcell, P. (2009a). *Income of Americans Aged 65 and Older, 1968 to 2008.* Washington, DC: Congressional Research Service.

Purcell, P. (2009b). *Older Workers: Employment and Retirement Trends.* Congressional Research Service. Available: http://www.aging.senate.gov/crs/pension34.pdf [July 2010].

Quinn, J., Cahill, K., and Giandrea, M. (2011). Early retirement: The dawn of a new era? *TIAA-CREF Policy Brief.* Available: http://www.tiaa-cref.org/institute/research/briefs/pb_earlyretirement0711.html [January 2012].

Rehkopf, D., Adler, N., and Rowe, J. (2011). *Socioeconomic, Racial/Ethnic and Functional Status Impacts on the Future U.S. Workforce.* Paper prepared for the National Research Council Committee on the Long-Run Macroeconomic Effects of the Aging U.S. Population.

Restuccia, D., and Vandenbroucke, G. (2011). *Explaining Educational Attainment Across Countries and Over Time.* Department of Economics, University of Toronto. Available: http://www.phil.frb.org/phil_mailing_list/research-and-data/events/2011/macroeconomics-across-time-and-space/papers/restuccia-vandenbroucke.pdf [November 2011].

Richardson, D.P. (2008). Trends in health care spending and health insurance. *TIAA-CREF Institute Trends and Issues*, December. Available: http://www.tiaa-crefinstitute.org/institute/research/trends_issues/ti_healthcaretrends_1208.html [January 2012].

Riley, W.B., and Chow, K.V. (1992). Asset allocation and individual risk aversion. *Financial Analysts Journal*, 48, 32-37.

Rubinstein, Y., and Weiss, Y. (2006). Post schooling wage growth: Investment, search and learning. In E.A. Hanushek and F. Welch (Eds.), *Handbook of the Economics of Education, Volume 1* (pp. 1-67). Chicago: Elsevier Science.

Salthouse, T.A. (1991). *Theoretical Perspectives in Cognitive Aging.* Hillsdale, NJ: Erlbaum.

Schieber, S. (2004). Retirement income adequacy: Good news or bad? *Benefits Quarterly*, Fourth Quarter, 27-39.

Schieber, S.J., and Shoven, J.B. (1999). *The Real Deal: The History and Future of Social Security.* New Haven, CT: Yale University Press.

Schoeni, R.F., Freedman, V.A., and Martin, L.G. (2008). Why is late-life disability declining? *Milbank Quarterly*, 86(1), 47-89.

Scholz, J.K., Seshadri, A., and Khitatrakun, S. (2006). Are Americans saving "optimally" for retirement? *Journal of Political Economy*, 144(4), 607-643.

Seeman, T.E., Merkin, S.S., Crimmins, E.M., and Karlamangla, A.S. (2010). Disability trends among older Americans: National health and nutrition examination surveys, 1988-1994 and 1999-2004. *American Journal of Public Health*, 100(1), 100-107.

Seshamani M., and Gray, A. (2004). Ageing and healthcare expenditures: The red herring argument revisited. *Health Economics*, 13(4), 303-314.

Shang, B., and Goldman, D. (2007). Does age or life expectancy better predict health care expenditures? *Health Economics*, 17(4), 487-501.

Short, K. (2011). The research supplemental poverty measure: 2010. *Current Population Reports P60-241.* Available: http://www.census.gov/prod/2011pubs/p60-241.pdf [February 2012].

Simonton, D.K. (1988). Age and outstanding achievement: What do we know after a century of research? *Psychological Bulletin*, 104, 251-267.

Simonton, D.K. (1991). Career landmarks in science: Individual differences and interdisciplinary contrasts. *Developmental Psychology*, 27, 119-130.

Skirbekk, V. (2004). Age and individual productivity: A literature survey. *Vienna Yearbook of Population Research*, 2, 133-153.

Skirbekk, V., Loichinger, E., and Weber, D. (2012). Variation in cognitive function as a refined approach to comparing aging across countries. *Proceedings of the National Academy of Sciences*, 109(3), 770-774.

Smith, S., Newhouse, J.P., and Freeland, M.S. (2009). Income, insurance, and technology: Why does health spending outpace economic growth? *Health Affairs*, 28(5), 1276-1284.

Social Security Administration (SSA). (2010a). *Annual Statistical Supplement, 2010*. Available: http://www.ssa.gov/policy/docs/statcomps/supplement/2010/6b.html#table6.b5 [July 2011].
SSA. (2010b). *Income of the Population 55 or Older, 2008*. SSA Publication No. 13-11871. Washington, DC: Social Security Administration.
SSA. (2011). *Projected Future Course for SSA Disability Programs*. Available: http://www.ssa.gov/policy/docs/chartbooks/disability_trends/sect06.html [January 2012].
Stearns, S.C., and Norton, E.C. (2004). Time to include time to death? The future healthcare expenditures predictions. *Health Economics*, 13(4), 315-327.
Stock, J.H., and Wise, D.A. (1990a). Pensions, the option value of work, and retirement. *Econometrica*, 58(5), 1151-1180.
Stock, J.H., and Wise, D.A. (1990b). The pension inducement to retire: An option value analysis. In D.A. Wise (Ed.), *Issues in the Economics of Aging*. Chicago: University of Chicago Press.
Takats, E. (2010). *Aging and Asset Prices*. BIS Working Papers 313. Basel, Switzerland: Bank for International Settlements.
Taylor, M.G. (2010). Capturing transitions and trajectories: The role of socioeconomic status in later life disability. *The Journals of Gerontology, Psychological Sciences and Social Sciences*, 65B(6), 733-743.
Technical Panel on Assumptions and Methods. (2011). *Report to the Social Security Advisory Board, September 2011*. Pre-publication copy available: http://www.ssab.gov/Publications/Financing/2011_Technical_Panel_Report_prepublicati on.pdf [November 2011].
The Economist. (2006). Baby boom and bust. Will share prices crash as baby-boomers sell their assets to pay for retirement? Print version May 11, 2006. Available: http://www.economist.com/node/6914086 [March 2012].
Toossi, M. (2006). A new look at long-term labor force projections to 2050. *Monthly Labor Review*, November, 19-39.
Toossi, M. (2009). Labor force projections to 2018: Older workers staying more active. *Monthly Labor Review*, November, 30-51.
Tuljapurkar, S., Li, N., and Boe, C. (2000). A universal pattern of mortality decline in the G7 countries. *Nature*, 405, 789-792.
United Kingdom Pension Commission. Various reports, archived and available: http://www.webarchive.org.uk/wayback/archive/20070802120000/http://www.pe nsionscommission.org.uk/index.html [May 2011].
United Nations. (2001). *Replacement Migration: Is It a Solution to Declining and Ageing Populations?* New York: United Nations.
United Nations. (2011). *World Population Prospects: The 2010 Revision*. New York: United Nations.
University of California, Berkeley, and Max Planck Institute for Demographic Research. (2011). *Human Mortality Database*. Available: http://www.mortality.org or www.humanmortality.de [October 2011].
U.S. Census Bureau. (2008). *2008 National Population Projections*. Available: http://www.census.gov/population/www/projections/2008projections.html [November 2011].
U.S. Census Bureau. (2012). *The 2012 Statistical Abstract*. Available: http://www.census.gov/compendia/statab/2012edition.html [January 2012].
U.S. Census Bureau. (Various years). *Annual Social and Economic Supplements. Current Population Survey*. Available: http://www.census.gov/hhes/www/poverty/data/incpovhlth/2009/pov09fig05.pdf.
Venti, S., and Wise, D.A. (2001). Choice, chance, and wealth dispersion at retirement. In S. Ogura, T. Tachibanaki, and D.A. Wise (Eds.), *Aging Issues in the United States and Japan* (pp. 25-64). Chicago: University of Chicago Press.

Verbrugge, L.M., and Jette, A.M. (1994). The disablement process. *Social Science and Medicine*, 38, 1-14.

Vere, J.P. (2007). "Having it all" no longer: Fertility, female labor supply, and the new life choices of generation X. *Demography*, 44(4), 821-828.

Verhaegen, P., and Salthouse, T.A. (1997). Meta-analyses of age-cognition relations in adulthood. Estimates of linear and nonlinear age effects and structural models. *Psychological Bulletin*, 122(3), 231-249.

Vincent, G.K., and Velkoff, V.A. (2010). The next four decades. The older population in the United States: 2010 to 2050. *Current Population Reports*, P25-1138. Washington, DC: U.S. Census Bureau.

Waldron, H. (2002). *Mortality Differentials by Race*. Social Security Administration Division of Economic Research Working Paper, December. Available: http://www.ssa.gov/policy/docs/workingpapers/wp99.pdf [February 2012].

Wang, H., and Hanna, S. (1997). Does risk tolerance decrease with age? *Financial Counseling and Planning*, 8(2), 27-31.

Watson Wyatt Worldwide. (2004). *Phased Retirement: Aligning Employer Programs with Worker Preferences*. Washington, DC: Watson Wyatt Worldwide.

Webb, A. (2009). *Should You Carry a Mortgage into Retirement?* Center for Retirement Research at Boston College, Brief 9-15. Available: http://crr.bc.edu/wp-content/uploads/2009/07/IB_9-15.pdf [January 2012].

Wee, C.C., Huskey, K.W., Ngo, L.H., Fowler-Brown, A., Leveille, S.G., Mittlemen, M.A., and McCarthy, E.P. (2011). Obesity, race and risk for death or functional decline among Medicare beneficiaries. *Annals of Internal Medicine*, 154, 645-655.

Wentworth, S.G., and Pattison, D. (2002). Income growth and future poverty rates of the aged. *Social Security Bulletin*, 64(3), 23-37.

White House Council on Women and Girls. (2011). *Women in America. Indicators of Social and Economic Well-being*. Available: http://www.whitehouse.gov/administration/eop/cwg/data-on-women [November 2011].

Wilmoth, J.R. (1997). In search of limits. In K.W. Wachter and C.E. Finch (Eds.), *Between Zeus and the Salmon: The Biodemography of Longevity* (pp. 38-64). Washington, DC: National Academy Press.

Wilmoth, J.R. (2001). How long can we live? A review essay. *Population and Development Review*, 27(4), 791-800.

Wilmoth, J.R., Boe, C., and Barbieri, M. (2010). Geographic differences in life expectancy at age 50 in the United States compared with other high income countries. In E.M. Crimmins, S.H. Preston, and B. Cohen (Eds.), *International Differences in Mortality at Older Ages: Dimensions and Sources* (pp. 333-366). National Research Council. Washington, DC: The National Academies Press.

Wolfe, E.N. (2006). *The Adequacy of Retirement Resources among the Soon-to-Retire, 1983-2001*. Levy Economics Institute Working Paper 472. Available: http://www.levyinstitute.org/pubs/wp_472.pdf [December 2011].

Wyatt, I.D., and Hecker, D.E. (2006). Occupational changes during the 20th century. *Monthly Labor Review*, March, 35-57.

Yakoboski, P.J. (2010). Retirees, annuitization and defined contribution plans. *TIAA-CREF Institute Trends and Issues*, April. Available: http://www.tiaa-crefinstitute.org/institute/research/trends_issues/ti_definedcontributions0410.html [December 2011].

Appendixes

Appendix A

Population and Related Projections Made by the Committee

Gretchen S. Donehower and Carl Boe

This appendix outlines the methods used to generate the population and labor force projections as well as summary measures and other indicators used in several chapters of this report. The projections were reviewed for accuracy and consistency by committee members and compared with results from other such projections. While the committee's projections were made to 2100, the report primarily discusses results through 2050. Given the high degree of uncertainty regarding variables such as future rates of return, productivity growth, international capital flows, and so on, the committee chose to limit its analysis and discussion to the next four decades.

POPULATION PROJECTIONS BY AGE AND SEX

The population projections used by the committee are based on intermediate-cost population projections prepared by the Social Security Administration (SSA) for its 2011 Trustees Report, with some important modifications. The committee thanks Felicitie Bell, Office of the Chief Actuary of the SSA, for her generosity in sharing projection details with it. The Social Security methods are summarized here briefly, but complete information on SSA projection methods and assumptions can be found at http://www.ssa.gov/oact/tr/2011/index.html (accessed June 24, 2011). The starting population is the 2008 estimated Social Security Area population[1]

---

[1] The Social Security Area population covers the U.S. Census population (residents of all 50 states and Washington, D.C., plus Armed Forces overseas) but adds a small group of potential Social Security beneficiaries who are not covered by the U.S. Census population. These persons

by sex and single year of age. This population is projected forward each year based on projected rates of fertility, mortality, and net migration. Net migration is immigrants coming into the population minus emigrants leaving the population.

The age-specific fertility rates used are the same as in the intermediate-cost SSA projections, with a minor adjustment for the years 2008 and 2009.[2] The age distribution of fertility is based on recent historical trends, while the overall level of fertility is assumed to decline gradually in the near term and remain constant at just below replacement level. Specifically, the observed total fertility rate is 2.09 children per woman in 2008 and is assumed to fall gradually to a constant level of 2.00 children per woman by 2035.

The main adjustment to the SSA projections is that the mortality rates used here are lower than those used in the intermediate-cost SSA projection. As described in Chapter 3, the committee agrees with the Social Security Advisory Board's Technical Panel on Assumptions and Methods (TPAM) that there will likely be faster future declines in mortality than reflected in the intermediate-cost SSA projections. This conclusion is based on an analysis of potential future trends in smoking and obesity (Technical Panel on Assumptions and Methods, 2011). The SSA projection assumes that average life expectancy by 2050 will be 82.2 years, whereas the committee projection assumes instead an additional 2.3 years of life on average, for a life expectancy of 84.5 years by 2050. This mirrors the TPAM conclusion. The corresponding lower age-specific mortality rates are found by searching for a mortality schedule that is between the SSA intermediate- and high-cost options and implies a life expectancy in 2050 of 84.5 years. The high-cost option assumes lower mortality than the intermediate and thus an average life expectancy of 84.8 years by 2050. The projection used here employs a mortality schedule that is a weighted average of the two SSA options such that the desired life expectancy in 2050 of 84.5 years is achieved.

This average is found by first defining a difference term $b_{x,s}$ for age x and sex s, which is the difference between the death rates $m_{x,s}$ for the high cost and intermediate cost:

$$b_{x,s} = \ln(m_{x,s}^{\text{high}}) - \ln(m_{x,s}^{\text{intermediate}})$$

---

are U.S. citizens living abroad, residents of U.S. territories, and noncitizens living abroad who are insured for future Social Security benefits. They usually comprise around 2 percent of the U.S. Census population. In the aggregate, the Census and Social Security Area population age and sex distributions are almost identical.

[2]Published rates for 2008 were multiplied by 0.99 and for 2009 by 1.01 to match more closely the predicted birth cohorts of the SSA projections and correct for inconsistencies introduced by interpolation to estimate January 1 populations from July 1 population estimates.

The new death rates that were used for these projections are

$$m_{x,s} = \exp\{\ln(m_{x,s}^{\text{intermediate}}) + kb_{x,s}\}$$

where k, which is the same for both sexes and constant over age, is found by a search program to achieve the desired average life expectancy of 84.5 years in 2050.

The SSA projection adds net migrants at each projection step based on a guess about the future trend of migration, legal and illegal combined, and the age and sex distribution of net migrants from recent history. The total number of net migrants in the SSA projections begins at only 35,000 in 2008 based on evidence that the recent economic downturn in the United States has discouraged a great deal of potential immigration and encouraged some emigration. The projected number of net migrants quickly rebounds to 1,250,000 by 2015 but then falls slowly but steadily to 1,025,000 by 2085. While the committee's projection uses the same age and sex distribution of net migration as in the SSA 2011 Trustees Report from 2008 to 2025, its trajectory for future migration is significantly higher than that of the SSA. As with future mortality, the committee believes that the future trajectory for net migration developed by the TPAM is more reasonable than the one currently used in intermediate SSA projections. Thus the committee adopted the TPAM migration schedule for 2026-2050, which assumes a constant rate of 3.2 net migrants for every 1,000 residents each year after 2025.

Given the rates of fertility, mortality, and net migration described above, the starting Social Security Area population of 2008 is projected forward in single-year steps of age and time for men and women separately using the cohort component method. The projection ends in the year 2100.[3] This projection was the baseline scenario of future change. Summary measures for fertility, life expectancy, and net migration appear in Table A-1. For several analyses reported in previous chapters, the rates of fertility, mortality, and net migration were modified to calculate population projections based on alternative scenarios of change. In these cases, the projections were exactly as described above, except for the alternative rates described in the scenario.

---

[3]The SSA 2011 Trustees Report only published projection results to year 2085 because it is charged with reporting a 75-year time horizon for Social Security finances. The demographic projections, however, are estimated internally to 2100.

TABLE A-1 Summary Measures of Demographic Assumptions for Baseline Projection, Selected Years 2008-2100

Year	Years of Life Expectancy			Total Fertility Rate (births per woman)	Net Migrants (millions)
	Men	Women	Combined		
2008	75.4	80.3	77.8	2.05	0.04
2009	75.6	80.4	77.9	2.04	0.84
2010	75.7	80.5	78.1	2.07	0.82
2015	76.9	81.3	79.0	2.05	1.25
2020	77.9	82.1	79.9	2.04	1.20
2025	78.8	82.9	80.8	2.02	1.14
2030	79.7	83.6	81.6	2.01	1.19
2035	80.5	84.3	82.4	2.00	1.23
2040	81.3	85.0	83.1	2.00	1.27
2045	82.1	85.7	83.8	2.00	1.31
2050	82.8	86.3	84.5	2.00	1.34
2055	83.5	86.9	85.1	2.00	1.38
2060	84.2	87.4	85.8	2.00	1.43
2065	84.8	88.0	86.3	2.00	1.47
2070	85.4	88.5	86.9	2.00	1.52
2075	86.0	89.0	87.4	2.00	1.57
2080	86.5	89.4	88.0	2.00	1.62
2085	87.1	89.9	88.5	2.00	1.67
2090	87.6	90.3	88.9	2.00	1.72
2095	88.1	90.7	89.4	2.00	1.78
2100	88.6	91.1	89.8	2.00	1.84

SOURCE: Committee calculations.

POPULATION PROJECTIONS BY RACE/ETHNIC GROUP

For some of the analyses, population projections by separate groups defined by race and ethnicity were of interest. The SSA does not take race or ethnicity into account when it makes projections, so data from the U.S. Census Bureau were used to break the SSA-based population projections into race/ethnic groups that are consistent with the main population projections used in this report. The committee thanks David Waddington, Ben Bolender, Christine Guarneri, and Donnette Willis of the Population Projections Branch of the U.S. Census Bureau for sharing data with it for the project.

Census Bureau projections are done based on the resident population by age, sex, race, and Hispanic origin. The set of projections published in 2008 was used here and can be found at http://www.census.gov/population/www/projections/2008projections.html (data first accessed May 31, 2011). These projections cover the years 2008 to 2050, so the committee extends the Census 2050 rates to the year 2100 to cover the full period of interest.

While the Census projections define many additional groups, only five groups were used in this work to avoid small numbers in groups defined by sex, single years of age, and race/ethnicity. The five race/ethnicity groups used were (1) Hispanic, (2) non-Hispanic white alone, (3) non-Hispanic black alone, (4) non-Hispanic Asian alone, and (5) non-Hispanic other. This last group includes non-Hispanic native Hawaiian and Pacific Islanders, American Indians and Alaska natives, and multiracial persons.

Census Bureau projected rates based on these five groups do not aggregate to the same rates as in the baseline single-group projection described in the preceding section. This is due both to the modifications in SSA rates made by the committee and to the different projection methods used by the Census Bureau and the SSA. To keep the projection by race/ethnic group consistent with the single-group projection, it was necessary to use the race/ethnic projections from Census to disaggregate the baseline projection rather than using Census rates by race/ethnic groups and projecting them directly.

This means that the starting population for the race/ethnic projections is not the starting population of the Census Bureau race/ethnic population projections. Instead, each age and sex group in the starting population for the single-group projection is broken down into the five race/ethnic groups based on the distribution in the Census Bureau population for that age and sex group.

Then, at each projection step, the total number of vital events (births, deaths, net migrants) for each age and sex group is estimated for the single-race projection and broken down into the five race/ethnic groups based on the distribution that would have occurred given the relative rates (of fertility, mortality, or net migration) from the Census Bureau race/ethnic population projections. In this way, the single-sex and race/ethnic projections are consistent with each other but the relative changes in the race/ethnic groups are consistent with the Census Bureau rates by race/ethnic group.

For example, say mortality rates for the single-group projection predicted 900 deaths to men aged 52 during the year, while the Census mortality rates by race/ethnic group projected 800 deaths across the five race/ethnic groups. The 900 single-group deaths would be multiplied by the race/ethnic distribution of the 800 deaths to get the race/ethnic distribution of the 900 deaths to men aged 52 during the year.

Finally, while the Census Bureau publishes mortality rates by each age/sex/race/ethnic group, this is not the case for fertility or net migration. Birth rates are published by race/ethnic group only, not age, so the projection assumes that the age distribution of fertility for all five race/ethnic groups is the same as the overall SSA age distribution of fertility. Net migration is published as counts by sex and race/ethnic group, so the projection assumes that the age distribution of male net migration is the same as the SSA age distribution of male net migrants for all five race/ethnic groups. Similarly for females, the SSA age distribution of female net migrants is used for all females across race/ethnic groups.

LABOR FORCE PROJECTIONS

The Bureau of Labor Statistics (BLS) usually projects the labor force only 10 years into the future. Occasionally, though, it extends those near-term projections to longer periods of time. The labor force projections in this report are based on labor force participation rates from a longer-term projection, one first produced in 2006 and later updated to a starting year of 2008. The method mainly takes historical trends within each age/sex/race/ethnic group and extrapolates them into the future, but with a logit transformation so that the future path is nonlinear. During the first part of the projection period, through 2020, changes in the labor force "are the result not only of compositional changes in the population, but also of changes in the detailed labor force participation rates of the various age, sex, race, and ethnic categories. [These] latter changes are based on the past labor force behavior of those categories and are often assumed to approach zero beyond a certain point in the projection horizon. Accordingly, changes in the aggregate labor force participation rate and in the labor force between 2020 and 2050 will reflect only changes in the age, sex, race, and ethnic composition of the population." (Toossi, 2006, p. 22) There is no economic model involved in the BLS projections, nor is there any attempt to include the effects of the business cycle.

The BLS data end in 2050, so the 2050 labor force participation rates were repeated to extend to a 2100 projection horizon. No estimates are provided for those younger than age 16, so their labor force participation rate is assumed to be zero. The details of the labor force projections can be found at http://www.bls.gov/opub/mlr/2006/11/art3full.pdf. (Data with projections through 2050 were accessed on July 11, 2011, but are no longer available on the BLS Web site.)

The BLS labor force participation rates are estimated by sex for single years of time, but for age the groups may span 2 years, 5 years, or more. To apply these rates to the population schedules by sex and single years of age, an interpolation method was used. A cubic spline was fitted to the cumulative counts of population and labor force, generating estimates of the total population and labor force at each age. The ratio of these produces labor force participation rates by single years of age that are completely consistent with the BLS age group rates but provide a smooth single-year-age schedule. These rates by sex and single year of age and time were then applied to the population projection described previously to get the total projected labor force by age and sex.

Note that the BLS labor force participation rates are based on a universe of the civilian noninstitutional population. They were applied here to a universe that includes noncivilians and the institutional population to avoid the need for estimating a further projection of future rates of military service and institutionalization by age, sex, and race/ethnic group. In the aggregate, the impact of the different population bases is very small.

The BLS does not include race/ethnicity in its labor force projections, so data from the March Current Population Survey (CPS) were used to estimate labor force participation rates by the same five race/ethnic groups discussed above. The CPS data were accessed through the Integrated Public Use Microdata Series facility, found at http://cps.ipums.org/cps/. Specifically, rates for the five groups from 2000 to 2011 were averaged together to estimate the labor force participation rates of the five groups within each age and sex group. Five-year age groups were initially estimated to reduce noise in the estimates, and then the same cumulative spline interpolation described above was applied to obtain a smooth single-year-of-age schedule. Then, a single multiplicative adjustment factor for each age-sex-year cell was computed so that the overall age-sex-year labor force participation rate was preserved; however, the race/ethnic groups had relative participation rates in the same ratios as the CPS rates by race/ethnicity for that age and sex.

SUPPORT RATIO ANALYSES

Calculating a support ratio requires two types of data: counts of population by age and per capita estimates of economic activity by age. The committee refers to the second item, the age schedules of per capita economic activity, as "age profiles." The National Transfer Accounts project has a fully developed methodology for estimating age profiles of economic activity for individuals by age from surveys and administrative data. Details on the methodology are available at the project Web site, www.ntaccounts.org, and in Mason and Lee (2011). Examples of age profiles for consumption and production appear in Figure A-1 for the United States in 2007. Details on the sources and methods for constructing U.S. age profiles are found in Lee, Donehower, and Miller (2011).

A support ratio (SR) is the ratio of aggregate age profiles weighted by population. In mathematical notation, let $c(x,t)$ and $yl(x,t)$ represent the consumption and labor income profiles, respectively, in Figure A-1 at each age x at time t. Let $n(x,t)$ be the number of persons age x in the population at time t. For a support ratio indicating the relative number of producers to consumers, the calculation is

$$SR(t) = \sum_{x=0}^{\varepsilon} yl(x,t)\, n(x,t) \,/\, \sum_{x=0}^{\varepsilon} c(x,t)\, n(x,t)$$

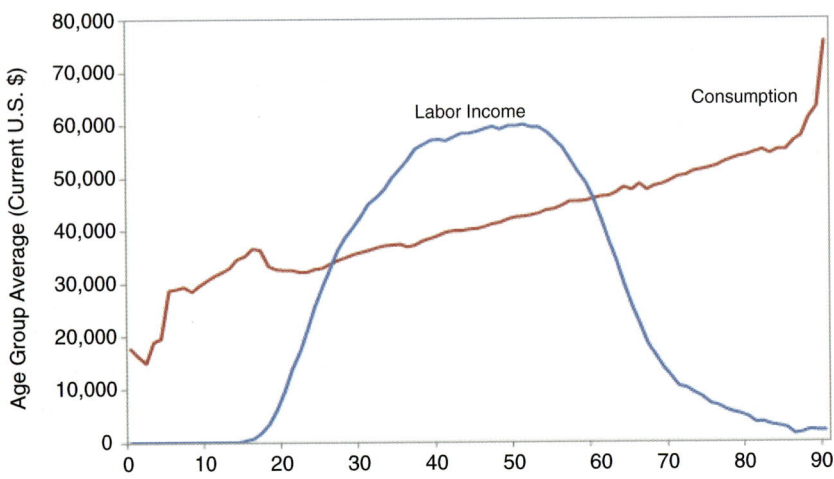

FIGURE A-1 U.S. per capita labor income and consumption, by single year of age, 2007. SOURCE: Committee calculations.

Similarly, a fiscal SR can be calculated substituting the age profile of taxes paid for labor income in the numerator and the age profile of government benefits received for consumption in the denominator.

The SR calculated for one time t in this way gives a snapshot of the aggregate balance between different pairs of age profiles at time t. If we combine the age profiles of a fixed time with a population projection, we can assess what will happen to the balance of age profiles, say labor income and consumption, over time if the age profiles remain fixed but the demography changes. For example, combining the age profiles shown in Figure A-1 with the U.S. population projection detailed in the first section allows generating a time series for t from 2007 to 2100:

$$SR(t) = \sum_{x=0}^{\varepsilon} yl(x,2007) \, n(x,t) / \sum_{x=0}^{\varepsilon} c(x,2007) \, n(x,t)$$

This analysis was done for other countries with age profiles calculated as part of the National Transfer Accounts project, using the age profiles calculated for a recent year and combining them with population counts from the United Nations World Population Prospects database, medium variant projections (http://esa.un.org/wpp/unpp/panel_population.htm).

Calculating a time series of SRs in this way shows how population aging affects the ratio of producers to consumers or taxpayers to beneficiaries over time. It indicates what will happen if age profiles are held constant and population changes.

Another type of analysis asks how age profiles would have to change to maintain the level of the SR in the face of population aging. This was done by taking the labor income curve and extending the peak value for an additional year of age. For example, using 2007 age profiles for the United States and the population projection developed for this report, the support ratio in the United States for 2007 was 0.78. The peak value of average labor income was about $60,000 for people aged 51. Given population aging, the SR in the following year fell to just under that in 2007. Instead of allowing the support ratio to fall in 2008, the committee imagines that the age profile of labor income stretches at age 51, repeating the $60,000 value for age 52. The rest of the age profile shifts to the right by 1 year. The old age 52 value is assigned to age 53, and so on. Then the support ratio for 2008 becomes 0.80. This is above the initial 2007 value, so we proceed to the next year. The support ratio for 2009 to 2014 with the labor income curve stretched by 1 year is still above 0.78, so no further adjustment is needed. In 2015, however, the support ratio with the 1-year labor income extension falls below the 0.78 value, so the labor income curve must be extended again. Now labor income's $60,000 peak value appears for ages 51, 52, and 53, and the original value for age 52 is assigned to age 54, for age 53 to age 55, and so on. Repeating this algorithm for the whole population projection gives an indication of roughly how many years retirement would have to be delayed on average to keep the SR from falling below its current level. This type of calculation can be made for other "thought experiments," such as how much taxes would have to rise to maintain the current fiscal SR.

A different but more straightforward calculation indicates how much consumption would have to fall to maintain the current SR if labor income stayed fixed. That figure is simply the unadjusted SR divided by the SR in the starting year.

INCOME-WEIGHTED POPULATION

The future impacts of population aging may be conditioned by the socioeconomic conditions of countries with different future aging trajectories. To include this variable in the analysis, estimates of future population age distributions were calculated based not just on counts of population by age, but also by weighted population counts by age—that is, weighted by the relative wealth of the country where each projected person resides.

To review the basic population-weighted calculation where each person counts equally, let $n(j,x,t)$ be the number of persons in country j of age x at time t. The global population age distribution, or the proportion of people in the world age q across all j countries at time t, is

$$\text{Global Population Age Distribution} = \sum_{j=1}^{J} n(j,q,t) / \sum_{j=1}^{J} \sum_{x=1}^{\varepsilon} n(j,x,t)$$

which is the global number of persons aged q at time t divided by the global population at time t.

Now we can add a differential weight to each person in the calculation, based on the per capita gross domestic product (GDP) of each country j at time t, or GDP(j,t):

$$\text{GDP-Weighted Global Population Age Distribution} = \sum_{j=1}^{J} \text{GDP}(j,t)\, n(j,q,t) \Big/ \sum_{j=1}^{J} \sum_{x=1}^{\varepsilon} \text{GDP}(j,t)\, n(j,x,t)$$

These analyses were done using several different data sources. The population by age and country were taken from the United Nations World Population Prospects database, medium variant projections for 2008, available at http://esa.un.org/wpp/unpp/panel_population.htm. Different GDP data were used to assess the robustness of the results to different data sources or scenarios.

One option was to use 2010 per capita GDP data for the entire projection period. The per capita GDP figures, measured in purchasing power parity-adjusted international dollars, came from the International Monetary Fund's (IMF's) World Economic Outlook database, the April 2011 version, available at http://www.imf.org/external/pubs/ft/weo/2011/01/weodata/download.aspx (accessed April 28, 2011).

Another option was to use per capita GDP figures for 2010 but multiply them by projected GDP growth rates to get a projected per capita GDP for each country. This was done using two different sources for the projected GDP growth rates. The first was the IMF World Economic Outlook database mentioned above, which has a projection of average annual growth from 2010 to 2016. This average annual rate was used to project each country's GDP out to 2050, which was then divided by its projected population to get its projected per capita GDP (all adjusted for purchasing power parity). The second source was the consulting firm PriceWaterhouseCoopers, which estimates GDP growth using reports on future economic opportunities. Projected rates from 2010 to 2050 for 22 countries covering over 80 percent of 2010 global economic output are available at http://www.pwc.com/en_GX/gx/world-2050/pdf/world-in-2050-jan-2011.pdf (accessed April 28, 2011). As with the IMF projections, these rates were used to grow GDP from observed 2010 levels, which were then divided by projected population to get the per capita figures (also adjusted for purchasing power parity). For those countries not included in the PriceWaterhouseCoopers report, IMF data were used but adjusted by the ratio of the average PriceWaterhouseCoopers growth estimates to the IMF growth estimates for the 22 countries with data from both sources.

A few disputed territories or small islands that did not have both population and GDP projection data were dropped from the analysis.

TOTAL NET WORTH

If net worth differs by age, then population aging will have an impact on total net worth and thus the pool of assets available to an economy to fund growth. To examine this possibility, the committee used data on the average net worth of families in the United States by the age of the family head. These data come from the 2007 wave of the Survey of Consumer Finances (SCF), reported in the Federal Reserve's February 2009 Bulletin (available at http://www.federalreserve.gov/pubs/bulletin/2009/pdf/scf09.pdf).

Let $NW(x,t)$ be the average net worth of a family with head age x at time t. In order to apply this family measure to individuals, the committee assumed that all assets are owned by the head of the family and that nonheads have no assets. When $NW(x,t)$ is multiplied by the headship rate $h(x,t)$, or the proportion of persons age x who are family heads at time t, the product is the average net worth of a person age x at time t.[4] The data on headship come from the 2007 March Supplement of the CPS. The CPS data were accessed through the Integrated Public Use Microdata Series facility found at http://cps.ipums.org/cps/.[5]

Finally, multiplying the average net worth per person in 2007, $NW(x,2007)h(x,2007)$, by the population schedule $n(x,t)$ gives the total net worth at time t. Dividing through by the total population gives the per capita amount:

$$\text{Per Capita Net Worth } (t) = \sum_{x=1}^{\varepsilon} NW(x, 2007)\, h(x, 2007)\, n(x,t) \Big/ \sum_{x=1}^{\varepsilon} n(x,t)$$

As with the other calculations in this report, the committee is interested in the change brought about by population aging. This formula gives some indication of that by showing what will happen to per capita net worth in the future if the age profile of net worth and headship remain constant but the population continues to age.

---

[4]Note that $NW(x,t)$ is the ratio of total net worth of families headed by those age x to the number of families headed by those age x. The headship rate $h(x,t)$ is the ratio of the number of families headed by those age x to the number of persons age x. Multiply these two quantities together and the family terms cancel, leaving a ratio of total net worth of families headed by those age x to the number of persons age x. This is per capita net worth if we assume that only family heads own the assets.

[5]The concept of family in the CPS is not exactly the same as that in the SCF, so the headship data used from the CPS are the headship rates for households, not families. Across the entire population, the differences in family and household headship are small, as most households contain only one family, by both the SCF and CPS definitions.

STOCHASTIC POPULATION PROJECTIONS

Stochastic forecasts of fertility and mortality rates by age and sex, together with initial population counts and a deterministic migration schedule, allow for the generation of stochastic population trajectories through time that reflect uncertainty or variation around a long-term trend. The stochastic population counts (denoted $N_{s,x,t}^{i}$, where the indices are sex (s), age (x), and time (t) and where i indicates a specific trajectory) in turn yield stochastic support ratios, SR_t^i.

The level of uncertainty is a function of the amount of natural variation in the historical vital rates and in the forecast uncertainties of mortality and fertility components. The methodology is that described in Lee and Tuljapurkar (1994), where the Lee-Carter model is used for both the mortality and fertility components.

Mortality

Stochastic mortality trajectories were generated following the coherent forecast technique of Li and Lee (2005), which is a Lee-Carter model. This coherent method lowers forecast uncertainty by grouping forecasts for 15 low-mortality countries. Inputs to the model are mortality rates for 1950-2007 from the Human Mortality Database (University of California, Berkeley, and Max Planck Institute for Demographic Research, 2011); output consists of 1,000 stochastic sex-age-time trajectories $M_{s,x,t}^{i}$ from the online LCfit program (available at http://simsoc.demog.berkeley.edu/). Each projection i is independent from projection $j \neq i$, and any life table functional such as e_0 may be computed from the set of underlying death rates by fixing the trajectory number, time, and sex. The median in 2050 of the 1,000 trajectories for combined-sex e_0 is close to 84.5, the target value from the baseline deterministic mortality projections in Table A-1.

The trajectories $M_{s,x,t}^{i}$ are "calibrated" so that the median of e_0 for each sex matches up with the baseline values in Table A-1. Specifically, multipliers $z_{s,t}$ near unity are calculated so that

$$\text{median } e_0\,(z_{s,t}\,M_{s,x,t}^{i}) = e_0\text{baseline}(s,t)$$

This affects the cloud of trajectories by changing the center while preserving the density of the cloud about the center.

Fertility

The fertility forecasts consist of simulations from a Lee-Carter model of age-specific fertility rates (ASFR), using data from the 2011 Trustees Re-

APPENDIX A

port of the Social Security Administration (http://www.ssa.gov/oact/tr/2011/index.html) and the small adjustments to data circa 2008 described earlier. The least-squares fit provided by the singular value decomposition of the 1917-2010 series of ASFR yields i trajectories:

$$\text{ASFR}_{x,t}^{i} = a_x + b_x K_t^i$$

where $a_x = \text{ASFR}_{x,2010}^{i}$ and $\Sigma |b_x| = 1$ and K_t^i is a constrained autoregressive moving average (1,1) process with autoregressive coefficient 0.9673 and moving average coefficient 0.5367. The process is constrained so that the long-run average total fertility rate is 2.0 (see Lee and Tuljapurkar, 1994, for further details).

Migration

Net migration flows into the population follow the assumptions used in the deterministic population projections by age and sex (see Table A-1). Each stochastic trajectory experiences the same migration pattern.

Population

A population trajectory i begins with the initial launch population by age and sex in 2009, $N_{s,x,2009}^{i}$. To bring this population to 2010, losses from death during the year and additions from new births are determined using rates $M_{s,x,2009}^{i}$ and $\text{ASFR}_{s,x,2009}^{i}$ applied to the population. Finally, immigrants are added according to the baseline schedule.

Support Ratio

The SR for the i th trajectory,

$$SR^i(t) = \sum_{x=0}^{t} yl(x,t) N^i(x,t) / \sum_{x=0}^{\varepsilon} c(x,t) N^i(x,t)$$

is calculated along the trajectory based on the stochastic population counts. The consumption schedule $c(x,t)$ is normalized so that the support ratio in 2007 is unity.

Appendix B

Biographical Sketches of Committee Members

Roger W. Ferguson, Jr. (*Co-chair*) is president and CEO of TIAA-CREF. Prior to holding this position, he was head of financial services for Swiss Re, chairman of Swiss Re America Holding Corporation, and a member of the company's executive committee. Before that, Dr. Ferguson served as vice chairman of the board of governors of the U.S. Federal Reserve System. He joined the Federal Reserve in 1997 and became vice chairman in 1999. He was a voting member of the Federal Open Market Committee, served as chairman of the Financial Stability Forum, and chaired Fed committees on banking supervision and regulation, payment system policy, and reserve bank oversight. In 2001, he led the Federal Reserve's immediate response to the terrorist attacks on September 11. Prior to joining the Federal Reserve Board, Dr. Ferguson was an associate and partner at McKinsey & Company from 1984 to 1997. From 1981 to 1984, he was an attorney at the New York City office of Davis Polk & Wardwell, where he worked on syndicated loans, public offerings, mergers and acquisitions, and new product development. Dr. Ferguson is a fellow of the American Academy of Arts and Sciences and a member of the Academy's Commission on the Humanities and Social Sciences. He is a member of President Obama's Council on Jobs and Competitiveness and served on its predecessor, the Economic Recovery Advisory Board. He is co-chair of the Committee on Economic Development, and he serves on the boards of International Flavors & Fragrances Inc. and Audax Health. He is also a board member of the American Council of Life Insurers, the Institute for Advanced Study, and Memorial Sloan-Kettering Cancer Center. He is a member of the Advisory Board of Brevan Howard Asset Management LLP, chairman of the Economic Club of New York, and a member of the Council on Foreign Relations, the Harvard University Visiting Committee for the Memorial Church, and the Group of Thirty. Dr. Ferguson has authored or coauthored numerous speeches, lectures, articles, and monographs, including "Lessons from Past Productivity Booms" (*Journal of Economic Perspectives*, 2004) and "International Financial Stability" (*Geneva Report*, 2007). He has also lectured on macroeconomics, monetary policy, and retirement policy at several major universities. He proposed the creation of the *International Journal of Central Banking*, which commenced publication in 2005 and now has more than 50 sponsoring institutions. Dr. Ferguson holds a B.A., a J.D., and a Ph.D. in economics, all from Harvard University.

Ronald Lee (*Co-chair*) is a professor of demography and the Jordan Family Professor of Economics at the University of California, Berkeley. He is the director of the Center on the Economics and Demography of Aging at the University of California, Berkeley, funded by the National Institute on Aging (NIA). He has taught courses in economic demography, population theory, population and economic development, demographic forecasting, population aging, indirect estimation, and research design, as well as a number of proseminars. His current research focuses on intergenerational transfers and population aging. He codirects with Andrew Mason the National Transfer Accounts project, which estimates intergenerational flows of resources through the public and private sectors in 37 collaborating countries. He also continues to work on modeling and forecasting demographic time series, and the solvency of social security systems. In addition, he works on the biological evolution of intergenerational transfers and sociality and the way these interact with the evolution of other aspects of life history. Dr. Lee's notable honors include the presidency of the Population Association of America (PAA), the PAA Mindel C. Sheps Award for research in mathematical demography, the PAA Irene B. Taeuber Award for outstanding contributions in the field of demography, and an honorary doctorate from Lund University, Sweden. He is an elected member of the National Academy of Sciences, the American Association for the Advancement of Science, the American Academy of Arts and Sciences, the American Philosophical Society, and a corresponding member of the British Academy. Dr. Lee has held NIA merit awards continuously since 1994. He holds an M.A. in demography from the University of California, Berkeley, and a Ph.D. in economics from Harvard University.

Alan J. Auerbach is Robert D. Burch Professor of Economics and Law at the University of California, Berkeley. He is also director of the Burch Center for Tax Policy and Public Finance. He served as an assistant, then associate, professor of economics at Harvard University, and as a professor of law and economics at the University of Pennsylvania. He has served as a research associate at the National Bureau of Economic Research and as the deputy chief of staff on the U.S. Joint Committee on Taxation. Dr. Auerbach was elected to the American Academy of Arts and Sciences in 1999. He has authored numerous articles, books, and reviews, was formerly editor of the *Journal of Economic Perspectives*, and is the founding editor of *American Economic Journal: Economic Policy*. He holds a B.A. in economics and mathematics from Yale University and a Ph.D. in economics from Harvard University.

Axel Boersch-Supan is a professor of macroeconomics and public policy and founding and executive director of the Mannheim Research Institute for the Economics of Aging at Mannheim University, Germany. He is a full-time member of the Max Planck Society and a codirector of the Max Planck Institute for Social Law and Social Policy in Munich. He is also a research associate at the National Bureau of Economic Research and adjunct researcher at the RAND Corporation. He is a member of the German National Academy of Sciences, the Berlin-Brandenburg Academy of Sciences, and the MacArthur Foundation Aging Societies Network. He was chairman of the Council of Advisors to the German Economics Ministry, has cochaired the German Pension Reform Commission, and was member of the German President's Commission on Demographic Change. Dr. Boersch-Supan has served as a consultant to many governments, the Organisation for Economic Co-operation and Development, and the World Bank. His current research focuses on household retirement and savings behavior, age and productivity, and the macroeconomic implications of global aging. He also directs the Survey of Health, Ageing and Retirement in Europe (SHARE), a longitudinal data collection effort to study the interaction of health, aging, and retirement processes in 20 countries, financed by the European Commission. He holds a Ph.D. from the Massachusetts Institute of Technology.

John Bongaarts is a vice president and Distinguished Scholar at The Population Council, where he has worked since 1973. His research focuses on a variety of population issues, including the determinants of fertility, population–environment relationships, the demographic impact of the AIDS epidemic, population aging, and population policy options in the developing world. Dr. Bongaarts is a member of the National Academy of Sciences, the Royal Dutch Academy of Sciences, and the Johns Hopkins Society of Scholars. He has received the Robert J. Lapham Award and the Mindel Sheps Award from the Population Association of America, and the Research Career Development Award from the National Institutes of Health. He holds an M.S. from the Eindhoven Institute of Technology, Netherlands, and a Ph.D. in physiology and biomedical engineering from the University of Illinois.

Susan M. Collins is the Joan and Sanford Weill Dean of Public Policy at the Ford School and a professor of public policy and economics at the University of Michigan. Before coming to Michigan, she was a professor of economics at Georgetown University and a senior fellow with the Brookings Institution, where she retains a nonresident affiliation. Her area of expertise is international economics, including issues in both macroeconomics and trade. Her recent work explores implications of increasing international economic integration as well as determinants of economic growth in industrial and developing countries. She has coauthored studies comparing growth experiences in China and India and examining challenges to growth in Puerto Rico. She is a research associate at the National Bureau of Economic Research, secretary/treasurer of the Executive Committee of the Association of Professional Schools of International Affairs (APSIA), and in 2006-2008 was an elected member of the American Economic Association (AEA) Executive Committee. Dr. Collins served as a senior staff economist on the President's Council of Economic Advisers during 1989-1990 and chaired the AEA Committee on the Status of Minority Groups during 1994-1998. She holds a B.A. in economics from Harvard University and a Ph.D. in economics from the Massachusetts Institute of Technology.

Charles M. Lucas heads his own firm, Osprey Point Consulting. He retired as corporate vice president and director of Market Risk Management at American International Group (AIG). Prior to joining AIG in 1996, he was the senior vice president and director of risk assessment and control at Republic National Bank of New York, where he headed the Risk Assessment and Control Department, reporting to the Risk Assessment Committee of the board of directors. Prior to joining Republic in late 1993, Dr. Lucas was senior vice president of the Federal Reserve Bank of New York (FRBNY), in charge of the international capital markets staff. He joined the Federal Reserve in 1968 as an economist in the Domestic Research Division, moving through a variety of posts until being appointed in 1974 as an officer of the FRBNY. He was granted a leave of absence in August 1978 to work with the International Monetary Fund on a technical assistance mission to the Central Bank of Ceylon (now Sri Lanka). Dr. Lucas has also consulted in monetary policy planning and implementation with Bank Indonesia, Bangladesh Bank, and the Bank of Morocco. He returned to the FRBNY in 1979, serving in a variety of positions culminating in senior vice president. Dr. Lucas is a member of the Advisory Group on the Financial Engineering Program at the Haas School of Business, University of California, Berkeley, a member of the Corporation, Woods Hole Oceanographic Institution, and a director of Algorithmics, Incorporated. He holds a B.A. and a Ph.D. in economics from the University of California, Berkeley.

Deborah J. Lucas is a professor of finance in the Sloan School of Management at the Massachusetts Institute of Technology. Dr. Lucas's recent research has focused on the problem of measuring and accounting for risk in the evaluation of federal financial obligations and defined benefit pension liabilities. She has published papers on a wide range of topics including the effect of idiosyncratic risk on asset prices and portfolio choice, dynamic models of corporate finance, monetary economics, and valuing federal financial guarantees. Dr. Lucas recently edited the National Bureau of Economic Research (NBER) book *Measuring and Managing Federal Financial Risk*. She is a research associate of the NBER and a member of the National Academy of Social Insurance. Past appointments include chief economist for the Congressional Budget Office; senior staff economist for the Council of Economic Advisers; member of the Social Security Technical Advisory Panel; and professor of finance at Northwestern University's Kellogg School of Management. She holds a B.A. in economics and applied mathematics, an M.A. in economics, and a Ph.D. in economics, all from the University of Chicago.

Olivia S. Mitchell is the International Foundation of Employee Benefit Plans Professor, professor of insurance/risk management and business economics/policy, and the executive director of the Pension Research Council, all at the Wharton School of the University of Pennsylvania. She also directs the Boettner Center on Pensions and Retirement Research, is a fellow of the Wharton Financial Institutions Center and the Leonard Davis Institute, and sits on the board of the Population Aging Research Center at the University. Concurrently Dr. Mitchell is a research associate at the National Bureau of Economic Research and a coinvestigator for the Health and Retirement Study at the University of Michigan. Dr. Mitchell's research and teaching focus on international private and public insurance, risk management, public finance, and compensation and pensions. Her extensive publications (24 books and more than 170 articles) analyze pensions and health care systems, wealth, health, work, well-being, and retirement. Her coauthored study on Social Security reform won the Paul Samuelson Award for Outstanding Writing on Lifelong Financial Security from TIAA-CREF and she also received the Premio Internazionale dell'Istituto Nazionale delle Assicurazioni (INA) from the Accademia Nazionale dei Lincei, Rome, Italy, ex aequo. Dr. Mitchell previously taught at Cornell University, and she has been a visiting scholar at Harvard University, the Goethe University of Frankfurt, Singapore Management University, and the University of New South Wales. She served on President Bush's Commission to Strengthen

Social Security and the U.S. Department of Labor's ERISA Advisory Council. She was a member of the board of Alexander and Alexander Services, Inc.; the National Academy of Social Insurance board; and the executive committee for the American Economic Association. She also cochaired the Technical Panel on Trends in Retirement Income and Saving for the Social Security Advisory Council and was a board member of the Committee on the Status of Women in the Economics Profession as well as the Government Accountability Office Advisory Board. Dr. Mitchell has spoken for many groups including the World Economic Forum, the International Monetary Fund, the Investment Company Institute, the International Foundation of Employee Benefit Plans, the White House Conference on Social Security, and the President's Economic Forum, and she has provided testimony to committees of the U.S. Congress, the U.K. Parliament, the Australian Parliament, and the Brazilian Senate. She holds a B.A. in economics from Harvard University and an M.A. and a Ph.D. in economics from the University of Wisconsin, Madison.

William D. Nordhaus is Sterling Professor of Economics at Yale University. He has been on the faculty of Yale University since 1967 and has been full professor of economics since 1973. He is on the research staff of the National Bureau of Economic Research and the Cowles Foundation for Research and has been a member and senior advisor of the Brookings Panel on Economic Activity, Washington, D.C., since 1972. Dr. Nordhaus is current or past editor of several scientific journals and has served on the executive committees of the American Economic Association and the Eastern Economic Association. He serves on the Congressional Budget Office Panel of Economic Experts and was the first chairman of the Advisory Committee for the Bureau of Economic Analysis. He has studied wage and price behavior, health economics, augmented national accounting, the political business cycle, and productivity. Dr. Nordhaus is a member of the National Academy of Sciences and a fellow of the American Academy of Arts and Sciences. His 1996 study of the economic history of lighting back to Babylonian times found that the measurement of long-term economic growth has been significantly underestimated. In 2004, he was awarded the Distinguished Fellow prize by the American Economic Association. From 1977 to 1979, he was a member of the President's Council of Economic Advisers. From 1986 to 1988, he served as the provost of Yale University. He is the author of many books, among them *Invention, Growth and Welfare, Is Growth Obsolete?, The Efficient Use of Energy Resources, Reforming Federal Regulation, Managing the Global Commons, Warming the World*, and (jointly with Paul Samuelson) the classic textbook *Economics*, whose nineteenth edition was published in 2009. He holds a B.A. and an M.A.

from Yale University and a Ph.D. in economics from the Massachusetts Institute of Technology.

James M. Poterba is the Mitsui Professor of Economics at the Massachusetts Institute of Technology. He is also president of the National Bureau of Economic Research and a fellow of both the American Academy of Arts and Sciences and the Econometric Society. He is the president-elect of the Eastern Economic Association, the past president of the National Tax Association, a former vice president of the American Economic Association, and a former director of the American Finance Association. Dr. Poterba's research focuses on how taxation affects the economic decisions of households and firms. His recent work has emphasized the effect of taxation on the financial behavior of households, particularly their saving and portfolio decisions. He has been especially interested in the analysis of tax-deferred retirement saving programs such as 401(k) plans and in the role of annuities in financing retirement consumption. Dr. Poterba served as a member of the President's Advisory Panel on Federal Tax Reform in 2005. He is a trustee of the College Retirement Equity Fund (CREF) and the Alfred P. Sloan Foundation. He edited the *Journal of Public Economics*, the leading international journal for research on taxation and government spending, between 1997 and 2006. He is a member of the advisory board of the *Journal of Wealth Management*. Dr. Poterba is a co-author of *The Role of Annuity Markets in Financing Retirement* (2001), and an editor or coeditor of *Global Warming: Economic Policy Responses* (1991), *International Comparisons of Household Saving* (1994), *Empirical Foundations of Household Taxation* (1996), *Fiscal Institutions and Fiscal Performance* (1999), and *Fiscal Reform in Colombia* (2005). He has been an Alfred P. Sloan Foundation fellow, a Batterymarch fellow, a fellow at the Center for Advanced Study in Behavioral Sciences, and a distinguished visiting fellow at the Hoover Institution at Stanford University. He holds a B.A. in economics from Harvard and a D.Phil. in economics from Oxford University.

John W. Rowe is a professor in the Department of Health Policy and Management at the Columbia University Mailman School of Public Health. From 2000 until late 2006, Dr. Rowe served as chairman and chief executive officer of Aetna, Inc., a leading national health care and benefits organization. From 1998 to 2000, Dr. Rowe served as president and chief executive officer of Mount Sinai NYU Health, one of the nation's largest academic health care organizations. From 1988 to 1998, prior to the Mount Sinai-NYU Health merger, Dr. Rowe was president of the Mount Sinai Hospital and the Mount Sinai School of Medicine in New York City. Before joining Mount Sinai, Dr. Rowe was a professor of medicine and the founding director of the Division on Aging at the Harvard Medical School, as well as chief of gerontology at Boston's Beth Israel Hospital. He has received many honors and awards for his research and health policy efforts regarding care of the elderly. He was director of the MacArthur Foundation Research Network on Successful Aging and currently leads the MacArthur Foundation's Research Network on an Aging Society. Dr. Rowe was elected a member of the Institute of Medicine, a fellow of the American Academy of Arts and Sciences, and a trustee of the Rockefeller Foundation and Lincoln Center Theater. He is currently serving as a member of the Roundtable on Value & Science-Driven Health Care. He holds a B.S. from Canisius College and an M.D. from the University of Rochester.

Louise M. Sheiner is a senior economist at the board of governors of the Federal Reserve System. She has also held positions as the deputy assistant secretary for economic policy at the U.S. Department of the Treasury, senior staff economist for the Council of Economic Advisers, and economist for the Joint Committee on Taxation. Dr. Sheiner's expertise covers a range of disciplines, including health, fiscal policy, public economics, and welfare. Her recent publications include *Should America Save for Its Old Age? Fiscal Policy, Population Aging, and National Saving*; *Generational Aspects of Medicare*; and *Demographics and Medical Care Spending: Standard and Non-Standard Effects*. She holds a B.A. in biology and a Ph.D. in economics, both from Harvard University.

David A. Wise is the John F. Stambaugh Professor of Political Economy at Harvard University's John F. Kennedy School of Government. His past research includes analysis of youth employment, the economics of education and schooling decisions, and methodological econometric work. His work now focuses on issues related to population aging, and he directs a large project on the economics of aging and health care at the National Bureau of Economic Research. His recent books and papers include *Social Security and Retirement Around the World*; *Frontiers in the Economics of Aging*; *Facing the Age Wave*; *Inquiries in the Economics of Aging*; *Social Security and Retirement Around the World: Micro-Estimation*; *The Transition to Personal Accounts and Increasing Retirement Wealth: Macro and Micro Evidence*; *Aging and Housing Equity: Another Look*; *Implications of Rising Personal Retirement Saving*; *The Taxation of Pensions: A Shelter Can Become a Trap*; *Utility Evaluation of Risk in Retirement Saving Accounts*; and *Analyses in the Economics of Aging*. He holds a B.A. in French from the University of Washington and an M.A. in statistics and a Ph.D. in economics from the University of California, Berkeley.